Nursing Diagnoses and Process in Psychiatric Mental Health Nursing

Gertrude K. McFarland, R.N., D.N.Sc.
Nurse Consultant, Division of Nursing
U.S.P.H.S., Health Resources and Services Administration
U.S. Department of Health and Human Services
Rockville, Maryland

Formerly Chief, Nursing Education Section
Psychiatric Clinical Nurse Specialist
Saint Elizabeths Hospital
National Institute of Mental Health
U.S. Department of Health and Human Services
Washington, D.C.

Evelyn L. Wasli, R.N. D.N.Sc.
Acting Associate Chief Nurse
Psychiatric Nursing Coordinator
Saint Elizabeths Hospital
National Institute of Mental Health
U.S. Department of Health and Human Services
Washington, D.C.

Formerly Associate Professor
School of Nursing
Columbia Union College
Takoma Park, Maryland

Nursing Diagnoses and Process in Psychiatric Mental Health Nursing

J. B. Lippincott Company   Philadelphia
London   Mexico City   New York   St. Louis   São Paulo   Sydney

The opinions expressed herein are those of the authors and do not necessarily reflect those of the US Department of Health and Human Services or the Health Resources and Services Administration or those of Saint Elizabeths Hospital, respectively.

Sponsoring Editor: Diana Intenzo
Manuscript Editor and Production Coordinator: Linda Fitzpatrick
Indexer: Nancy Newman
Designer: Anne O'Donnell
Production Supervisor: J. Corey Gray
Compositor: American–Stratford Graphic Services, Inc.
Printer/Binder: R. R. Donnelley & Sons Co.

6 5 4

Library of Congress Cataloging in Publication Data

McFarland, Gertrude K., 1941–
    Nursing diagnoses and process in psychiatric mental health nursing.

    Includes bibliographies and index.
    1. Psychiatric nursing.   2. Mental illness—Diagnosis.
I. Wasli, Evelyn L.   II. Title.   [DNLM: 1. Mental
Disorders—diagnosis.   2. Nursing Process.
3. Psychiatric Nursing.   WY 160 M478n]
RC440.M32   1986   616.89′075   85-15878
ISBN 0-397-54598-3

The authors and publisher have exerted every effort to ensure that drug selection and dosage set forth in this text are in accord with current recommendations and practice at the time of publication. However, in view of ongoing research, changes in government regulations, and the constant flow of information relating to drug therapy and drug reactions, the reader is urged to check the package insert for each drug for any change in indications and dosage and for added warnings and precautions. This is particularly important when the recommended agent is a new or infrequently employed drug.

Consultants

Robert Keisling, M.D.
Medical Director/Mental Health Services Administrator
District of Columbia Government
Washington, D.C.

Assistant Professor of Psychiatry
George Washington University Medical Center
Washington, D.C.

Vallory Lathrop, R.N., D.N.SC., F.A.A.N.
Deputy Director for Nursing
Saint Elizabeths Hospital
National Institute of Mental Health
Washington, D.C.

Preface

While practicing in an era of cost-containment, every nurse should have a goal of providing the highest quality of nursing care. This text contains the concepts and principles essential to caring for clients who have behavioral problems. Content is presented in as practical a format as possible so that nurses can be guided in caring for the client who is experiencing behavioral or mental health problems in whatever setting care is being rendered.

The authors have presented information that is necessary for the understanding of mental health and mental illness. The major schools of psychiatric thought are concisely described. Techniques and concepts useful in developing the therapeutic nurse–patient relationship and in facilitating communication are illustrated with examples. The nursing process is introduced, a systems theory–based conceptual model for the practice of psychiatric nursing is illustrated, and a chapter on psychosocial assessment is provided.

The authors have selected those nursing diagnoses from the most current North American Nursing Diagnoses Association (NANDA) listing that are most relevant to the psychosocial care of clients. (The entire official NANDA listing of nursing diagnoses is provided in the text.) Based on extensive literature review, research, clinical observation and practice, and colleague input, a number of nursing diagnoses have been added where there appear to be gaps in the listing developed by NANDA to date. Provided for each nursing diagnosis presented are a definition, general principles, etiology, defining characteristics, strategies for nursing assessment, suggested goals and nursing interventions, content on health education and health promotion, and evaluation criteria. Separate chapters cover selected nursing interventions and knowledge about selected psychiatric disorders and related psychiatric treatment modalities.

The reader may note that throughout this book *he* has been used to refer to the patient and *she* has been used to refer to the nurse. The authors would like to emphasize that this distinction has been made only to preserve the readability of the text; thus, *he* refers to both male and female patients, and *she* refers to both male and female nurses.

The authors envision that as these nursing diagnoses continue to be tested and utilized in clinical practice, additional knowledge will be generated that will provide input to NANDA's ongoing development work.

The authors wish to acknowledge their families—Al McFarland, Ph.D., and parents John and Emma Ramseier; Arne Wasli and sons Kevin and Eric—for their support and patience during the preparation of this project.

Our appreciation is also extended to all those nurses who are working diligently to develop, clinically utilize, and research nursing diagnoses.

Contents

Nursing Diagnoses and Process in Psychiatric Mental Health Nursing

1
Concepts of Mental Health and Mental Illness

Definitions

1. *Mental health*—"A state of being, relative rather than absolute. The best indices of mental health are simultaneous success at working, loving, and creating with the capacity for mature and flexible resolution of conflicts between instincts, conscience, important other people, and reality."[1]
2. *Jahoda's six cardinal aspects of mental health*—These aspects include a positive attitude toward self, active growth and development toward self-actualization, integration, autonomy and independence from social influences, accurate perception of reality, environmental mastery.
3. *Roger's process of self-actualization*—The person engaging in the process exhibits openness to experience, lack of defensiveness, accuracy in symbolization, congruency, flexibility, unconditional self-regard, creative adaptation, effective reality testing, harmony with others.
4. *Mental illness*—"An illness with psychologic or behavioral manifestations and/or impairment in functioning due to a social, psychologic, genetic, physical/chemical, or biologic disturbance. The disorder is not limited to relations between people and society. The illness is characterized by symptoms and/or impairment in functioning."[2,3] Some common indicators of mental illness are depression, feelings of anxiety that are not proportionate to a possible cause, physical complaints having no organic cause, any sudden change of behavior or mood, unreasonable and unrealistic expectations of self or others, and failure to achieve potential.
5. *Insanity*—A legal concept describing a mental disturbance affecting a person with the consequence that he is not criminally responsible for an act. Rules and criteria for insanity are set by legal process.
   a. Mc Naughten Rule declared a person insane and not responsible for the criminal act if he had a disease of the mind that impaired his ability to distinguish right from wrong.
   b. Durham Rule said that the accused is not guilty if the unlawful act was done as a product of mental illness or deficit.
   c. American Law Institute test stated that if the defendant has a mental

1

disease or deficit and consequently lacks the capacity to appreciate the criminality of his behavior or to conform his behavior to the law, he is not responsible for the criminal act.

Statistics Regarding Mental Illness and Treatment

1. General health service system and not the specialty mental health services system provides most of the care.
2. Schizophrenia and depression cause people to seek mental health services frequently.
3. Approximately 20% of the population experiences a mental disorder.[4]
4. Phobias, alcohol abuse or dependence, dysthymia, and major depression are the most common disorders.[5]
5. 3727 facilities were providing mental services in 1980. Since 1975, there has been a decrease in number of state and county mental hospitals and clinics (they number 691, or 18.5% of total). Community Mental Health Centers (CMHC), which are federally funded, have increased (they number 923, or 24.8% of total).[6]
6. 274,713 inpatient beds were available in 1980. Since 1975, there has been a decrease in the number of beds per 100,000 population from 264 to 124; most of the reduction has been in state and county mental hospitals. There has not been a corresponding increase in number of other inpatient beds.[7]
7. 139,546 resident patients were in state and county mental hospitals in 1980. Since 1975, there has been a 62% decrease in the number of resident patients; the number of elderly and those with organic brain syndromes also has decreased in the hospitals.[8]
8. 380,371 additions to state and county hospitals in 1970 were made. The most frequent diagnoses were schizophrenia (36%), alcohol and drug abuse or dependence (27.3%), and organic brain syndrome (5.3%).[9]
9. 1648 facilities offered day treatment services in 1980. Since 1975, the services have doubled.[10]
10. 2,634,727 outpatient additions in 1979 were found. This number has doubled since 1975. CMHCs showed the most additions, with 47% of the total number.[11]
11. 5% of registered nurses identify their area of clinical practice as psychiatric/mental health nursing. One third of these nurses have education at baccalaureate level or beyond.[12]
12. Approximately 1,000,000 people in the United States are homeless mentally ill, accounting for approximately 50% of the homeless population in this country. They consist of migrants, refugees, drug abusers, individuals with severe personality disorders, and people who are displaced, unemployed, and severely or chronically mentally ill.[13]

Causal and Relationship Factors in Mental Illness

1. Increasingly, the complex interchanges occurring in the nervous system are being studied and biological explanations of mental disorder are being accepted.
2. Generally, there is a lack of definitive causal factors in mental illness.

However, several factors have been shown to have a relationship to the occurrence of mental illness.

3. *Physiological factors* include defective genes, disturbance in neurotransmission, activity of endorphins, disturbances in immune system, hormone imbalance, abnormal blood factors, malnutrition, vitamin deficiencies, low blood sugar, sensory deprivation, and sleep and dream deprivation.
4. *Psychological factors* include mental attachment and deprivation, sibling position, parental behavior and child-rearing practices, double-bind process in communication, conflict, stress, and coping styles.
5. *Sociocultural and spiritual factors* include age, sex, race, marital status, occupation, education, economic status, social class, religious beliefs and values, migration, roles, ethnic mores, lack of participation in the community, lack of social support system, overcrowding, rapid social change, and availability of and impediments within health care systems.

Neurobiological Approach

Emphasizes a scientific approach, study of the nervous system, to explain and treat mental disorders. *Illness* is defined as a disturbance in the neurobiological system.

A. Theoretical basis: genetic studies

1. Children of schizophrenic parents have an increased risk of schizophrenia, regardless of whether they are raised by the parent with schizophrenia or by another person. Empirical studies support this finding.
2. Abnormal sensitivity to acetylcholine was found in manic-depressive patients and relatives who are or were patients with emotional disorders. Empirical studies support this finding.
3. *Diathesis stress theory*—Offers an explanation that the genetic disease produces an intrauterine metabolic disorder that causes changes in the central nervous system. The infant has problems in sensing and in perceiving and constructing his world and is thus more vulnerable to environmental stress.
4. *Monogenic bioamine theory*—Genetic disorder that produces an abnormal metabolite that affects the arousal system, making the world appear new and confusing and the symptoms of schizophrenia appear.
5. *Defective hedonic capacity theory*—There is a genetic impairment of the capacity to experience pleasure. The infant is further hampered by his inadequate pain/pleasure response in learning adaptive behavior.

B. Theoretical basis: neurotransmitters

1. Each neuron receives information through its many dendrites from thousands of other axons of neurons. Consequently, each neuron sends messages by its network of axons. The gap between the axon of one neuron and the dendrite of another neuron is the synapse, and the transaction occurring is the synaptic transmission.
2. Chemical substances called neurotransmitters are active in the synapse. The neurotransmitter is released from the endings of the axon. Other neurons are specifically sensitive to the chemical and dendrites respond.

3. The transmitters produce an excitatory or inhibitory effect at the synapse. One neuron has many synapses, with excitatory forces firing the neuron and inhibitory forces decreasing the firing. An imbalance of these forces may result in aggressiveness, rage, or lethargy.
4. Thousands of these chemical reactions are occurring at any one time and are the biological basis for thinking and feeling.
5. Characteristics of the neurotransmitter are
   a. Synthesis and storage of substance in neuron.
   b. Release of substance upon stimulation of neuron.
   c. Termination of activity by enzymes and uptake process.
6. The cell bodies of neurons containing certain transmitters—norepinephrine, dopamine, and serotonin—have been located in brainstem, and their pathways extending to the brain and spinal cord have been identified by histochemical fluorescence method. Further study of the pathways or tracts will explain seemingly unrelated symptoms.
7. Currently, the number of known transmitters is about 100. Some of the more well-known neurotransmitters are discussed subsequently.

C. Well-known neurotransmitters
1. Acetylcholine acts at approximately 5% to 10% of the synapses in the brain. Nerve–voluntary muscle messages and many autonomic nervous system messages are involved.
2. Norepinephrine
   a. The hypothalamus is the area that contains the most norepinephrine, but even there only 5% of synapses are affected. It is a catecholamine neurotransmitter that affects the sympathetic nerves of the autonomic nervous system, assisting the body to respond in emergencies. Examples are vasoconstriction, increase in heart rate, and increase in secretions of glands.
   b. Norepinephrine transmitter defect is one of the causes of depression. A tricyclic antidepressant, desipramine, inhibits the uptake of norepinephrine and relieves depression.
3. Dopamine
   a. Acts as a catecholamine transmitter, with most activity in the corpus striatum, which involves motor behavior.
   b. When the mechanism does not function, symptoms of Parkinson's disease—tremors and rigidity—appear.
   c. Drugs such as haldol and thorazine prevent dopamine from reacting with receptor molecules. In schizophrenia, there is an excessive amount of dopamine and an extreme sensitivity to it. This has provided support for the dopamine hypothesis of schizophrenia.
   d. Another drug, amphetamine, acts to release dopamine. Overdoses of amphetamine will produce symptoms that resemble those of schizophrenia.
   e. Lithium decreases the synthesis of catecholamines, dopamine, norepinephrine, and epinephrine, thus creating an antimanic action.
4. Serotonin acts as the raphe nuclei of the brainstem and has a role in the

sleep-wakefulness cycle. Psychotic drugs change the activity of these neurons.

5. Gamma-aminobutyric acid (GABA) acts as an inhibitor in approximately 25% to 40% of the brain synapses. Antianxiety drugs such as diazepam (Valium) enhance the action of GABA and thereby reduce anxiety.

6. Enkephalins and endorphins

   a. These are peptides (chains of amino acids) affecting neurons that are sensitive to opiates. Sites of concentration of the neurons are entrances of sensory nerves to the spinal cord, the periaqueductal gray area of brain, the solitary tract in the brainstem, and certain areas of the limbic system.

   b. They help explain the effects of acupuncture and hypnosis, pain transmission, depression of the respiratory system in opiate overdose, and euphoria caused by opiates. Other effects on drinking behavior, memory, and sexual behavior in females are being studied.

7. Monamine assists in the degradation of dopamine, norepinephrine, and serotonin at the synapse. Drugs inhibiting the action of monamine oxidase have an antidepressant effect.

D. Therapy

Diagnostic aids such as CT scans, EEGs, laboratory studies, radiographs, history of present illness, history of familial incidences of disorders, physical examination, and behavior observations are used to determine areas of dysfunction. Drugs that effect change in the neurobiological system are prescribed, and changes are monitored. There is some evidence that people with psychiatric disorders do not receive adequate drug treatment.[14]

Stress-Adaptation Approach

Emphasizes the role of stress in the increased incidence of illness. Illness is viewed as a human reaction pattern to stress or maladaptation.

A. Theoretical basis

1. Risk factors are associated with the development of mental disorder. Various writers continue to identify these risk factors, which include prematurity, poor diet, chromosomal disorders, accidents, and racial discrimination.

2. Life events that are stressors and contribute to development of crises include death of a spouse, divorce, and marital separation. There remains controversy of how stress mechanisms affect a person. If a person receives adequate support, the risk of illness is less.

3. Crisis exists when a person is unable to cope with a threat and experiences an increase in anxiety; he tries other coping mechanisms and the problem is resolved. If the problem is not resolved, the anxiety increases and a variety of symptoms can emerge, such as suicidal and homicidal thoughts, somatic symptoms, confusion, depression, isolation, and nonproductivity. Crises can be divided into three groups: maturational (*e.g.,* transition into

retirement), situational (*e.g.,* loss of a job), and adventitious (*e.g.,* earthquake).
4. Competence of a person in adapting to crisis affects adaptation process.
   a. A person makes a cognitive appraisal of the stressor. A situation can be viewed as a challenge by some, a catastrophe by others, and so on.
   b. Many coping behaviors, mechanisms, and strategies exist and are classified in various ways.
   c. Vaillant offers a hierarchy of ego defenses based on the Grant Study of Adult Development.[15]
      (1) Psychotic mechanisms: denial, distortion, delusional projection.
      (2) Immature ego defenses: fantasy, projection, passive aggression, hypochondriasis, acting out.
      (3) Neurotic ego defenses: intellectualization, repression, displacement, dissociation, reaction formation.
      (4) Mature ego defenses: sublimation, altruism, suppression, humor, anticipation.
5. The presence of a social support assists a person in problem-solving and offers sustenance during a crisis period.

B. Therapy

Focus is on establishing a working relationship with the client, problem identification and steps in resolution, support of coping strategies, enhancement of self-esteem, anticipatory guidance, and preventive interventions (*e.g.,* assisting a mother in parenting techniques). For further discussion, see the section on ineffective individual coping in Chapter 4.

Psychodynamic Approach

Emphasizes the influences of intrapsychic forces on observable behavior. *Illness* is defined in terms of behavior disorders that originate in conflicts occurring before 6 years of age among the id, ego, superego, and/or environment. Anxiety is then experienced as a result of these conflicts. Excessive use of mental defense mechanisms leads to serious behavioral disturbances.

A. Theoretical basis
1. Freud is recognized as the founder of the psychoanalytic school of thought.
2. Psychic activity is influenced by two drives: sexual and aggressive.
3. The psyche is divided into levels of consciousness.
   a. *Conscious*—The awareness of self and environment that occurs when a person is awake.
   b. *Preconscious*—Contains memories and thoughts that are easily recalled.
   c. *Unconscious*—Contains memories and thoughts that ordinarily do not enter consciousness.
4. Structural aspects of the psyche are
   a. *Id*—The part containing instinctual drives and impulses. The ego and superego develop from the id.

(1) *Pleasure principle*—The id seeks immediate release from tension or pleasure and avoids displeasure without regard for consequences.

(2) *Primary process thinking*—Mental activity of the id characterized by a collapse of time periods and by images mistaken for reality, occurring naturally in infants and during dreams and in some mental illnesses.

b. *Ego*—The part that assists the psyche in relating to the environment through such functions as memory and thinking and in resolving psyche conflicts. One of the more important functions is reality testing (the ego's function in sorting perceptions coming from the id and from the environment). Its primary growth period is 6 months to 3 years of age. It is the "I."

(1) *Reality principle*—States that the ego tends to delay satisfaction by accommodation to situational factors.

(2) *Secondary process thinking*—Mental activity of the ego characterized by reason, logic, and differentiating among people, situations, and things.

c. *Superego*—The part that evaluates thought and actions, rewarding the good and punishing the bad.

5. *Anxiety*—An automatic response occurring when the psyche is flooded with uncontrollable stimulation.

a. *Signal anxiety, or reality anxiety*—A type of anxiety produced by the ego in anticipation of danger, such as loss of a loved one or disapproval of superego.

b. *Moral anxiety*—Type of anxiety from overwhelming feelings of guilt or shame about an act or thought.

c. *Neurotic anxiety*—Type of anxiety in which impulses from the id, such as aggressive or sexual impulses, threaten to overpower the ego.

B. Psychosexual stages of development

These stages are crucial because they are periods during which unconscious conflicts among id, ego, and superego develop. Fixation, or arrest of development, at any stage may occur as a result of excessive gratification or deprivation.

1. *Oral stage* (birth to 1½ years)

a. The infant obtains relief from biological and psychological tensions through his mouth and lips.

b. Learns to depend on external objects.

c. Sucks, swallows, takes in, bites, chews, spits, and cries.

d. Experiences a warm, trusting, and dependent pattern of relating.

e. Gratifies needs and begins to delay immediate satisfaction.

f. Ego development begins primarily through the process of identification.

g. Problems and/or traits related to oral stage: over-dependency, clinging behavior, pessimism, optimism, narcissism (self-love), "world-owes-me-a-living" attitudes, alcoholism, smoking, overeating, drug addiction, refusal to eat, vomiting, gullibility.

2. *Anal stage* (1½ to 3 years)
   a. The infant achieves control over anal sphincter and gives up some of his control as he experiences toilet training.
   b. He and his parents are involved in issues of control over defecation.
      (1) He may give the feces as a gift or keep them or expel them violently.
      (2) He may control the time of defecation or do what he wants with the feces.
      (3) He may relinquish his control or comply with the control imposed.
   c. The sense of "I" becomes well developed.
   d. Problems and/or traits related to anal stage: compliance, defiance, perfectionism, obsessive-compulsiveness, antagonism, negativism, sadomasochism (pleasure from inflicting pain on others or self), procrastination, miserliness, stuttering, phobias, compulsions, constipation, bedwetting, overconformity, competitiveness, generosity, creativity, possessiveness.
3. *Phallic stage* (3 to 6 years)
   a. Child experiences the genitals, particularly the penis, as the main source of pleasurable sensation and interest.
   b. Parents are vital in the process of developing sexual identity.
   c. *Oedipus complex*—Describes the emotional attachment of boy for mother and ambivalent feelings toward father. The boy fears retaliation and possible loss of penis (*castration fear*) and he has wishes of killing father.
   d. *Electra complex*—Describes a girl's wishes for penis of father and hopes to take the place of mother, whom she blames for not having penis.
   e. The complex is resolved by girl or boy in the identification of the child with the parent of the same sex.
   f. The superego is strengthened as the child accepts the standards of the parent.
   g. Problems and/or traits related to phallic stage: homosexuality, transsexuality, problems with authority, overinvolvement in being sexually attractive.
4. *Latency stage* (6 to 12 years)
   a. Child experiences a quiet period during which the sexual drive is dormant.
   b. Sexual and aggressive drives are channeled into school activities, play, and work.
   c. Relationships are mostly with peers of same sex.
   d. Problems noted in latency stage: delinquency, rebelliousness, tics, restlessness, hysteria, anxiety states, anorexia.
5. *Genital stage* (12 years to adulthood)
   a. The person experiences onset of puberty, renewed interest in sexual activity, and conflicts that were unresolved in past developmental stages.
   b. He learns to develop mature relationships with males and females.
   c. He begins to stop depending on parents.

d. Problems arising in genital stage can include conflicts, character disorders, and other mental disorders.

C. Defense mechanisms

Mental processes used by the ego to reduce anxiety and conflict by modifying, distorting, or rejecting reality. The most frequently used defense mechanisms include

1. *Repression*—Major response used to keep painful thoughts, feelings, and impulses from consciousness.
2. *Denial*—Response acknowledges no awareness of a painful event.
3. *Reaction formation*—Response expresses feelings opposite to those being experienced.
4. *Projection*—Response ascribes to another person or object the unacceptable thoughts and feelings.
5. *Rationalization*—Response justifies behavior by an attempt to explain it logically.
6. *Undoing*—Response cancels the effect of another response just made.
7. *Displacement*—Response is misdirected from original person or object to safer target.
8. *Sublimation*—Response partially substitutes socially acceptable activities for unacceptable impulses.
9. *Regression*—Response in which person deals with anxiety by behaving at a level more appropriate to an earlier age.
10. *Identification*—Response by which the actions and feelings of a person are the same as those of a significant other.
11. *Introjection*—Response in which an aspect of behavior or thought of another is taken into the ego structure.
12. *Isolation*—Response in which person blocks the feeling associated with an unpleasant, threatening situation or thought.
13. *Suppression*—Response that is not unconscious and deliberately forces certain ideas from thought and action.

D. Therapy

1. *Psychoanalysis* is an intense relationship with a psychiatrist for a period of time for the purpose of helping the person establish conscious control of affect and behavior.
2. Through dream analysis, free association, interpretation, analysis of resistance and *transference* (ascribing to the psychiatrist the thoughts and feelings associated with parents or other important people), and neutrality, the therapist assists the patient in reducing the anxiety associated with thought.
3. Conflicts are brought into awareness and thus resolved.

Interpersonal Approach

Emphasizes the importance of interpersonal relationships and communication on behavior. *Behavior disorders* are a result of patterns of avoidance, use of substitutive processes, and experiences with significant adults.

A. Theoretical basis

1. Sullivan is noted for interpersonal theory of psychiatry.
2. *Satisfaction* is achieved through interaction to obtain relief from tension from biological drives or needs.
3. *Security* is achieved when basic needs are satisfied in relationship to a mothering person without the presence of anxiety.
4. *Self system* develops from the dynamic interplay of the basic needs and the interpersonal process to achieve satisfaction and security and avoid or decrease anxiety.
   a. Modes of experiencing describe one's perception and thoughts.
      (1) *Prototaxic mode*—Person identifies with the whole world; thoughts and responses are undifferentiated.
      (2) *Parataxic mode*—Person recognizes that things go together, but there is no logic. Things are put together only because one event occurs and is followed by another.
      (3) *Syntaxic mode*—Person is able to use logic in explaining events.
   b. Person appraises himself through significant others' reactions and organizes the appraisals in terms of
      (1) Bad me—Acts that result in anxiety.
      (2) Good me—Acts that cause no anxiety.
      (3) Not me—Acts that are totally disapproved; severe anxiety is experienced.

B. Stages of growth and development

Reflect emphasis of interpersonal approach.

1. Infancy—Lasts until the appearance of speech, which enables infant to change environment.
2. Childhood—Lasts to emergence of need for peers.
3. Juvenile—Lasts to need for close relationship.
4. Preadolescence—Lasts to puberty and beginning interest in opposite sex.
5. Early adolescence—Lasts to development of relationships with opposite sex.
6. Late adolescence—Lasts to the establishment of stable love relationship with another.

C. Anxiety

1. First develops as infant experiences tension or insecurity of mother.
2. Later is experienced whenever a threat of disapproval from a significant person occurs.
3. Avoidance behaviors develop to deal with anxiety:
   a. Physically avoiding the situation.
   b. Changing the interaction in the situation.
   c. Using selective inattention, which is the process the person employs to not attend to that which causes anxiety.
   d. Using substitutive processes in which person dissociates certain aspects of interpersonal system. The term *security operations* also is used to describe these processes; these are similar to the defense mechanisms described by Freud.

D. Therapy

1. Therapist is a participant observer and not a neutral object.
2. *Elucidation* is a principle that states that a behavior change can occur when one can identify, conceptualize, and evaluate his behavior.
3. Focus of interview is on exploring the avoidance behaviors, anxiety experiences, and the interpersonal context in which the avoidance behaviors and anxiety occur.

Ego Development Approach

Emphasizes the development of ego identity throughout the life span; developed by Erikson. *Illness* is characterized by problems with self, relationships, or society that may cause extension of the developmental period. Behavioral disorders result from unresolved conflicts during the stages of the life cycle.

A. Theoretical basis

1. Human beings progress through a series of eight psychosocial developmental stages.
2. The growth plan is governed by both social experiences and innate capacities, the epigenetic principle.
3. In each developmental stage, the potential exists for the person to develop a new task that serves as a building block for subsequent stages.
   Physical and psychosocial hazards may thwart the person from achieving the task central to a given developmental stage that negatively affects subsequent developmental stages and may lead to maladaptive behavioral patterns.

B. Erikson's eight developmental stages

1. *Infancy* (birth to 18 months)
   a. During this stage, the infant learns to *trust* self and others, provided his needs have been met in a consistent and satisfying manner.
   b. Confidence, realistic trust, hope, optimism, and the ability to form relationships in later life stem from such an attitude of trust.
   c. Subject to hazards such as mistreatment, the infant may develop *mistrust,* later reflected in hostility, suspiciousness, and a general feeling of dissatisfaction.
2. *Early childhood* (18 months to 3 years)
   a. In this stage, *autonomy* results from reassuring, constructively guided experiences in which the child is allowed to exercise self-control of his behavior without being subjected to experiences beyond his capabilities.
   b. Socially acceptable behaviors of holding and letting go, on which toilet training focuses during this stage, become generalized to other aspects of living.
   c. The development of autonomy leads to self-control without loss of self-esteem, a sense of pride and good will, the ability to initiate activities yet be cooperative, and appropriate generosity and withholding.
   d. Difficulties, such as from external overcontrol, can lead to *shame and*

doubt (*i.e.,* feelings of being exposed, lack of a belief in being able to control one's life, and a lack of self-worth).

3. *Late childhood* (3 to 5 years)
   a. The child develops *initiative,* the ability to undertake and plan tasks, the pleasure of being active, and the experience of a sense of purpose.
   b. Pleasure in attack and conquest aid in developing sexual identity and roles.
   c. Initiative is controlled by a developing conscience. The person grows to develop and strives to utilize his potentials in a socially appropriate manner.
   d. *Guilt,* accompanied by self-restriction and denial, can result from an unsuccessful negotiation of this stage. The person fails to develop his potential.

4. *School age* (6 to 12 years)
   a. The major task is *industry,* characterized by involvement in the world, construction and planning, development of relationships with peers, development of specific skills, and identification with admired others.
   b. A sense of competence and the pleasure of diligence develops.
   c. *Inferiority,* the feeling that one is unworthy and inadequate, can result from hindrances.

5. *Adolescence* (12 to 20 years)
   a. The developmental task is *identity,* a confident sense of self, commitment to a career, and finding one's place in society.
   b. Successful resolution leads to the ability to work toward long-term goals, self-esteem, and emotional stability.
   c. The danger is *role* confusion, characterized by feelings of confusion, lack of confidence, indecision, alienation, and possibly acting-out behavior.
   d. Unsuccessful resolution may require the adult to spend life-long energies attempting to resolve remaining conflicts.

6. *Young adulthood* (18 to 25 years)
   a. *Intimacy* is the major developmental task. The person develops the ability to love, to develop commitments to other persons, and to enter true mutual relationships.
   b. *Isolation* is the danger. The person remains distant from others, withdraws, enters into superficial relationships, or develops prejudices.

7. *Adulthood* (28 to 65 years)
   a. *Generativity* is the task. The adult becomes responsible for guiding children or for the creation and development of productive and constructive tasks.
   b. Failure leads to *stagnation,* personal impoverishment, and self-indulgence.

8. *Old age* (65 years to death)
   a. The last stage is characterized by feelings of acceptance, importance, and self-worth about the value of one's life, *integrity.*
   b. *Despair,* the negative outcome of this stage, is the sense of loss, a feeling of life's meaninglessness, and the feeling that life's goals have not been achieved and that it is too late to start over.

C. Therapy

Focus is on establishing trust not obtained early in life and helping patient gain insight into unconscious motivations, thus reducing anxiety.

Behaviorist Approach

Emphasizes observable and measurable behavioral processes. *Maladaptive behavior* can be classified as behavior excess, behavioral deficit, distortion of reinforcing stimuli, distortion of discrimination stimuli, and aversive behavior.

A. Theoretical basis

1. Watson, Pavlov, and Skinner contributed to the development of the behaviorist school of thought.
2. Two schools of thought have developed.
   a. *Behaviorism*—All behavior follows learning principles; therefore, behavior may become maladaptive but is not considered abnormal.
      (1) *Respondent conditioning*—Concept that states that a specific stimulus elicits a certain response.
      (2) *Operant conditioning*—Concept that states that behavior responses are influenced by what follows the response.
      (3) *Reinforcement*—Concept that states that a behavior response can be influenced by positive and negative rewards.
   b. *Cognitive behaviorism*—Behavior is influenced by cognition independently of the stimulus.
      (1) Important variables determining behavior include plans, beliefs, expectancies, encodings, and competencies.
      (2) Feelings are believed to follow thoughts.

B. Therapy

1. *Functional analysis* is analysis of the manifest behavior.
   a. What behaviors are problematic?
   b. Under what conditions does the behavior occur?
   c. What are the positive reinforcers?
   d. What are the negative reinforcers?
   e. What are the effective behaviors that could be used as substitutes or as reinforcers?
2. Techniques frequently used in behavioral therapy are systematic desensitization, flooding, implosion, positive reinforcement, programs such as assertiveness training, relaxation exercises, token economy, and sex therapy.
3. Cognitive therapy focuses on changing the internal contingencies, such as expectancies, distortions, self-injunctions, self-reproaches, and sequence of thoughts, to effect a behavior change.
4. Techniques in cognitive therapy include verbal probing, reality testing, thought substitution, role playing, self-monitoring, assignment of tasks, use of humor, and reflection.

Humanistic-Existential Approach

Emphasizes the holistic view of man, his individuality and intrinsic worth, the importance of experiencing the present, and the personal meanings of experience. According to Rogers, Maslow, and Frank, abnormal behavior is a consequence of the following:

Rogers—An incongruence exists between one's self-image and experience.

Maslow—Basic needs are not satisfied (air, food, water, safety, love, belonging, self-actualization).

Frank—Lack of meaning of life may result in illness.

A. Theoretical basis: Rogers
1. *Self* is a central concept because one's evaluation of life is related to views of the self: Who am I? What I can do? What am I able to do? What do I want to be? Man strives for self-actualization.
2. Incongruence can develop between the ideal self and the real self and/or reality. This causes dissatisfaction, anxiety, and activation of a self-defense mechanism.
3. Continuous feedback about behavior is being given to child by others. These experiences are integrated, denied, or accepted as truth by the child, thus affecting the self.
4. The importance of accepting one's feelings and not denying them and of recognizing one's own values and beliefs and not generally accepting the values of others is stressed.

B. Therapy

Therapist demonstrates unconditional positive self-regard (genuine acceptance), empathetic understanding (ability to perceive another's world), correctness, and congruence to assist patient in exploring his uniqueness and worth.

Family Approach

Differing conceptual views of family theory and family therapy exist. There is no accepted typology or diagnostic view of families.

A. Structural framework
1. Minuchin views the family as a social system with structure and organization in which the individual lives and responds. Transactional patterns develop that control the interaction and behavior of family members.
2. Maladaption is noted in the transactional patterns (*i.e.,* disengagement with no or minimal contact among the family members and enmeshment with an overinvolvement between and/or among members).
3. Therapy is directed toward initiating change in the family structure by clarifying boundaries, rules, and expectations.

B. Interactional framework: Satir and Haley
1. The double bind theory offers a way to view the development of dysfunction in a family system. Its characteristics are as follows:

a. The individual is in an important relationship that involves being able to understand what is communicated.
b. The other person in the relationship is communicating two orders of messages and they are contradictory.
c. The individual is unable to make a comment about either order of the messages and therefore is in a double bind.
2. Dysfunctional communication is produced by denying, rejecting, or disqualifying the relationship aspect as the message aspects of the communication; by differing punctuation in the interactions between two persons, which results in greater and greater differences; and by having symmetrical or rigid interaction patterns.
3. Problems are viewed as consequences of using a solution that obviously is not working. Mishandling occurs as
a. steps are not taken and action is needed;
b. steps are taken and no action is needed; or
c. steps are taken at every level of communication.
4. Therapy is directed toward change in the individual interaction patterns in the family system (*e.g.*, Satir) and/or change in the structure or transaction pattern (*e.g.*, Haley) by setting goals, giving tasks, symptom prescription, advertising symptoms, reframing behavior, and so on.

C. Bowen system theory

Presents a conceptualization of the emotional system over several generations. Emphasizes variables of anxiety and level of integration and their influence on the family system. Illness is viewed as an aspect of human adaptation in which a person experiences a level of undifferentiation resulting from the transmission of low levels of differentiation from past generations.

1. Theoretical basis
a. *Sibling position*—Personality characteristics are related to sibling position (10 have been identified) and provide predictive data.
b. *Triangles*—The basic unit of the emotional system (*i.e.*, a twosome and an outsider). When tension is experienced, each person will attempt to obtain the outside position. If the tension increases, one of the persons will triangle another; a larger and larger interlocking system is thus formed.
c. *Family projection process*—Anxiety is experienced by the mother, who may respond by becoming sensitive to the child and overconcerned. Mother's overattachment to the child is supported by the father. Child becomes anxious, demanding, and unable to function alone. Schizophrenia may develop following several generations of lower levels of differentiation as a result of the family projection process.
d. *Multigenerational transmission process*—The family projection process involves multiple generations, with one child in each generation becoming less differentiated and less able to function.
e. *Emotional cut-off*—Concept describes the process of separation from parents as people attempt to resolve the emotional attachments. The more

intense the cut-off from parents, the more likely that a person and his children will have similar problems in life.

  f. *Differentiation*—Concept is related to a state of being and to the process of becoming more responsible for self at emotional and intellectual levels. Profiles are developed for different levels of differentiation.

  g. *Nuclear family emotional system*—Patterns of functioning of mother, father, and children are identified. Major patterns include marital conflict, dysfunction in one spouse, projection of problems to a child, and/or a combination of these patterns.

  h. *Societal regression*—When a society is exposed to chronic anxiety, it responds with emotionality to relieve the anxiety; thus, functioning regresses. An example of regression response is overuse of drugs in society.

2. Therapy
  a. Focuses on reducing reactivity and increasing one's differentiation.
  b. Expression of feelings is not encouraged or interpreted, but person is assisted in thinking about processes.
  c. Exploration of family's past history is encouraged.
  d. Re-establishment of contact with family is supported.
  e. Therapist uses his skill to remain out of the interlocking triangles, thereby increasing flexibility and ability to decrease anxiety.

REFERENCES

1. Werner A et al (eds): Subcommittee of the Joint Commission on Public Affairs. A Psychiatric glossary, 5th ed, p 89. Washington DC, American Psychiatric Association, 1980
2. Ibid
3. American Psychiatric Association: Diagnostic and Statistical Manual of Mental Disorders (DSM 111), 3rd. Washington, DC, American Psychiatric Association, 1980
4. Myers JK et al: Six-month prevalence of psychiatric disorders in three communities, 1980–1982. Arch Gen Psychiatry 41 (10): 906, 1984
5. Ibid
6. Taube CA, Barrett SA (eds): Mental Health, United States, 1983 DHHS Publication No. (ADM)83-1275, p 10. Rockville, MD, The National Institute of Mental Health, 1983
7. Ibid, p 15
8. Ibid, p 34
9. Ibid, pp 31–32
10. Ibid, p 13
11. Ibid, p 27
12. Ibid, p 99
13. Bachrach LL: The homeless mentally ill and mental health services: An analytical review of the literature. In Lamb HR (ed): The homeless mentally ill. A task force report of the American Psychiatric Association, pp 20–21. Washington DC, American Psychiatric Association, 1984
14. Uhlenhutt et al: Symposium checklist syndrome in the general population. Arch Gen Psychiatry 40(11): 167–173, 1983
15. Vaillant E: Adaptation to Life. Boston, Little, Brown, 1977

2
Therapeutic Relationship

ELEMENTS OF THE NURSE–PATIENT RELATIONSHIP

The One-to-One Nurse–Patient Relationship

Definition and characteristics include:

1. Focusing attention on the patient and his emotional and behavioral concerns through a mutually defined professional relationship.
2. Using goal-directed therapeutic communication, including active listening, in order to foster exploration of problem areas, learning, change, and personal growth. Includes a series of nurse–patient interactions occurring over time.
3. Can range from brief counseling to more lengthy forms of treatment as individual nurse psychotherapy.

Phases of the Nurse–Patient Relationship

A. Phase I (beginning, or orientation, phase)

1. Patient uses primarily cognitive words and phrases—for example, when describing personal history, patient recounts primarily factual material.
2. Patient will often reach a point at which he will state that he has nothing more to say.
    a. For therapeutic progress, patient must move beyond this plateau into the affective domain and into Phase II of the relationship.
    b. To assist him in moving into the affective domain, focus on an identified cognitive theme that is linked with affective material.
3. Nurse therapist becomes acquainted with patient. The patient is assessed, and nursing diagnoses are formulated.
4. A mutually agreed upon contract for the one-to-one nurse–patient relationship is established.
    a. The nurse therapist's role and responsibilities in the one-to-one nurse–patient relationship are explained.
    b. The overall purpose of the one-to-one nurse–patient relationship is described.
    c. Initial, mutually defined behavioral goals are identified.
    d. The place, time, and length of the meeting are agreed upon.
    e. The actual or tentative length of the entire therapy is stated.

    f. Arrangements are made to deal with missed appointments.

    g. The responsibilities of the patient in the one-to-one nurse–patient relationship are discussed.

5. Of great importance is the formation of a working relationship with the patient.

    a. The patient begins to demonstrate a sense of confidence in—and liking for—the nurse therapist.

    b. The nurse therapist senses an ability "of making contact" with patient and an ability of being able to facilitate change and growth.

6. Discuss confidentiality of information shared by patient.

    a. Inform patient that progress in therapy will be reported to health care team members in general terms, with confidentiality of specific information maintained, except that

    b. Information about harmfulness to self or others will be shared with appropriate professional staff.

    c. Written progress reports may be shared prior to being placed on the patient's record.

7. Build trusting relationship by maintaining the stipulations of the contract and informing the patient of any changes, such as unavoidable absences.

B. Phase II (middle, or working, phase)

1. Phase in which patient discusses his problems and feelings and in which behavioral change and growth occur.

2. Affective material will dominate. Patient will use cognitive words and phrases to describe or emphasize material from affective domain.

3. Attend to frequency of affective word or words used and to behavioral trends and patterns described.

4. Encourage expression and analysis of emotional concerns and self-defeating behavioral patterns and trends.

    a. Mutually determine the behavioral dynamics of the patient: Explore origin, operation, and consequences of behavioral patterns.

    b. Facilitate patient's own assessment of self-defeating behavioral patterns.

5. Be aware of the possibility of resistance occurring.

    a. Behavioral manifestations of patient can include rejection, avoidance, denial, hostility, and reaching a plateau in therapy.

6. Facilitate resolution of emotional conflicts, reduction in self-defeating behavioral patterns, and attainment of the mutually defined behavioral goals of the patient.

    a. Identify forces with patient that hinder behavioral change.

    b. Facilitate problem-solving strategies to formulate behavioral alternatives and to select a behavioral alternative for testing.

    c. Create atmosphere in which the testing of new behaviors can readily occur and any associated anxiety can be worked through.

C. Phase III (termination, or resolution, phase)

1. The patient makes increasing use of cognitive words and themes in relation to future planning.

2. Patient responses to the actual termination with the nurse therapist are variable and are related to prior termination experiences, type of treatment, present problems, and personality.

   Reactions to impending loss can include grief, sadness, displacement, reaction formation, dependency, or frank hostility.

3. Interventions or tasks to be achieved in termination include the following:
   a. Assist patient to identify his responses to impending loss of therapist.
   b. Encourage patient to express feelings.
   c. Assist patient to work through and resolve his feelings about the impending separation from the therapist.
   d. Encourage patient to explore and evaluate his total experience in the one-to-one nurse–patient relationship.
   e. Give feedback to patient on his accomplishments and areas for further growth.
   f. Help patient tolerate the discomfort involved in termination.
   g. Mutually determine exact termination date.
   h. Encourage patient's emotional investment in others significant to him.
   i. Assist patient in planning for the future.

4. To facilitate termination and closure of relationship in a mutually planned, satisfying manner, instruct patient to
   a. Spend some time (at least a half hour) alone and without interruptions.
   b. Think about the relationship with the nurse therapist during the entire course of therapy.
   c. Stay with the feelings that are generated as long as needed.
   d. Imagine and practice how he wants the last session to be, until the last session is satisfying for him.
   e. Actually share thoughts, feelings, and fantasies with nurse in the therapy session. (The nurse therapist will also have gone through the preceding process and will share her thoughts and feelings.)

DEVELOPING A THERAPEUTIC RELATIONSHIP
Develop Effective Communication Skills
A. Definition and elements

1. *Communication*—A dynamic, complex, constantly changing process that occurs over time in which human beings send and receive verbal and nonverbal messages in order to understand and to be understood by others, adapt to the environment, and transfer ideas to another.
2. It is impossible not to communicate, because all behavior communicates something.
3. Communication includes
   a. Content aspect of message—Verbal message
   b. Relationship aspect of message—Verbal and/or nonverbal aspect of message about the relationship between the sender and the receiver.
      Nonverbal communication can qualify or disqualify verbal message.
4. Elements of communication include
   a. Sender—Transmits message.

    b. Message—Meaning that is communicated, intentionally or unintentionally.

    c. Code, channel, or media—The way in which a message is sent.

    d. Receiver—Recipient of message.

    e. Response of feedback—Behavior of receiver (verbal and nonverbal) in relation to message received.

B. Types of communication

1. Verbal—Use of written or spoken words, or
2. Nonverbal—Use of facial expression; eye contact; posture; bodily movements; touch; appearance and dress; pitch, rate, and volume of voice; gestures.
3. Digital—The verbal mode of communication, or
4. Analogic—The nonverbal mode of communication including the context.
5. Symmetrical—Communication characterized by equality in the right to initiate communication, to criticize, and to offer advice; or
6. Complementary—Communication characterized by one person giving and the other receiving in the interaction.

C. Factors affecting communication

1. Culture, customs, education, social background, physical attributes, mental well-being, body image, self-esteem, intellectual ability, and past experiences of the participants.
2. Channel, language, and words used to transmit message.
3. Context in which communication occurs.
4. Perceptions, feelings, thoughts, and motivations of receiver and sender prior to communication.
5. Nature of the relationship between sender and receiver.
6. Intentions or goals of sender.
7. Self-concept or self-perception of sender and receiver.
8. Anxiety or stress level of sender or receiver.
9. Sensory organ impairment or physical disorder interfering with mechanical ability to produce sound.
10. Discrepancies between the sender's and receiver's punctuation of the communication sequence of events—that is, the particular aspect of the communication on which each focuses—can affect the relationship.

D. Communication techniques

1. Understanding response—A response that conveys sincere effort to understand how the patient views his world, his experiences, and the meaning he attaches to his experiences.
2. Open-ended questions—Questions that present the patient with options for response other than just answering "yes" or "no."
    a. Avoid closed questions—Questions in which the nurse implies what answer is expected.
    b. Questioning can be useful in obtaining information, clarification, and offering assistance.

3. Reflection—Letting the patient know through feedback what he has overtly or covertly said or the feelings that he has conveyed. Use the same key words used by patient.
4. Active listening—Listening characterized by attending to patient's communications (not on own personal responses to be made), interpreting what is communicated, and responding selectively.
   a. Communicate concern, caring, and understanding. "Pick up on" feelings and needs expressed verbally and nonverbally.
   b. In responding selectively, use communication techniques as reflection, summarizing, and so on.
   c. After communicating understanding, use problem-solving approach to help patient explore alternatives.
   d. Use silence constructively and appropriately.
5. Seeking validation—Requesting feedback from patient to check understanding and interpretation of his communication or of his perceptions.
6. Sharing observation—Verbalizing what is observed about a patient's behavior; for example, "You appear rather sad."
7. Clarifying—Requesting feedback to make certain that patient's communications are accurately understood; for example, "By telling me . . . do you mean . . . ?" or "To whom are you referring when you say 'they'?"
8. Picking up on themes expressed—Providing feedback on ideas or feelings repetitively expressed, such as, "You seem to be feeling that your family can't be trusted." Avoid switching conversation to superficial topics.
9. Restating—Repeating a main thought, using words much like those used by the patient in order to encourage expansion.
10. Encouraging verbalization—Verbal and nonverbal means to assist patient to keep talking, such as "Go on" or "You were saying?" or nodding head.
11. Focusing—Asking questions or using other communication techniques to help patient stick to important subject matter or theme.
12. Feedback—Describing some aspect of patient's communication and its impact on the receiver.
13. Summarizing—Giving patient feedback on general content and theme of conversation in a condensed version.
14. Confrontation—Describing discrepancies in behavior of patient and encouraging exploration.

E. Examples of causes of communication breakdown or distortion
1. Unintelligible messages—Using terms the patient does not understand, especially psychiatric or medical terminology or jargon.
2. Incomplete messages—Assuming that the patient already has the knowledge and therefore leaving the patient's questions unanswered.
3. Inadvertent messages—Unintentionally transmitting a message, as by giving too much detail, which the patient then misinterprets.
4. Omitted messages—Failing to explain something the patient should know.
5. Contradictory messages—Transmitting a message in which the verbal

and nonverbal aspects are contradictory, or several different staff members giving different messages to the patient.

6. Unfulfilled messages—Making promises that are not kept.
7. Failure to listen actively.
8. Failure to interpret message accurately.
9. Failure to focus on patient's concerns.
10. Ineffective or inappropriate reassurance.
11. Lecturing, moralizing, pep talks.
12. Switching topic of conversation to superficial aspects.
13. Judgmental attitude, prejudice, stereotyping.
14. Stress perceived or faced by nurse in work situation.
15. High level of fear and anxiety patient may have about his illness and its treatment. (Items 1 through 14 can increase patient's anxiety.)

Develop and Improve Self-Awareness

1. Develop awareness of own verbal and nonverbal communication patterns.
2. Recognize, explore origin, and attempt to work through stereotyping, prejudices, and negative attitudes.
3. Develop awareness of own cultural and subcultural values and customs and their influence on personal behavior as well as on one's own perception and interpretation of another's behavior.
4. Identify common personal stressors and typical behavioral responses.
5. Identify and increase own adaptive coping patterns in response to stress.
6. Identify and develop constructive personal ethical values in relation to care of the adult psychiatric patient and health care in general.
7. Validate perceptions and interpretations of patient's behavior with patient or with professional colleague as indicated.
8. Examine own motives, feelings, and behavior.
   a. Develop self-acceptance, self-esteem, and self-respect.
   b. Develop ability to differentiate clearly between own feelings and those belonging to the patient.
   c. Recognize, accept, and analyze origin of negative feelings.
9. Seek qualified supervision as needed, especially when providing one-to-one nurse therapy.
10. Operate on facts rather than on assumptions or misperceptions.
11. Identify awareness of anxiety developed in self during a nurse–patient interaction and seek to gain information about the patient's anxiety level, using self as guide.

Develop Trust

Trust—A sense of confidence and security in the reliability of oneself and others.

1. Be consistently truthful.
2. Offer patient clear understanding of purpose of nurse–patient relationship or one-to-one nurse therapy
3. Be consistent, reliable, and open.

4. Demonstrate interest in, and commitment to, patient over a period of time.
5. Consistently communicate trustworthiness and credibility.
6. Be sensitive to patient's needs and his being.
7. Give information as needed by patient. Do not try to control patient.
8. Create interpersonal relationship in which patient can freely communicate his feelings, needs, and problems.
9. Communicate a warm, positive regard for patient.
10. Don't make promises unless they can be kept.
11. Try to respond to reasonable requests.

Be Congruent

Congruency—an expression of consistency between actual feelings, thoughts, verbalizations, and behavior.
1. Be natural, spontaneous, real, open, sincere, and nondefensive.
2. Admit own errors to patient, when appropriate.
3. Communicate negative feelings to patient if
   a. They are truly generated by patient, not from one's own past.
   b. The patient is capable of distinguishing the feedback to an aspect of his behavior and not to his total being.
   c. It can be done within the context of a therapeutic objective.
4. Share own personal reactions and feelings with patient if this serves a therapeutic purpose.
   a. Avoid constant and total disclosure of feelings.
   b. Express negative feelings to patient in a nondestructive way that encourages further discussion.
5. Be as natural and spontaneous as possible in the use of therapeutic interventions. Avoid artificial, mechanical use of interpersonal techniques.

Use Personal Self-Disclosure Appropriately

1. Patients' levels of self-disclosure have been positively correlated with their ability to deal with their illness.
2. If the nurse or patient discloses self at a certain level in the relationship, the other person tends to respond with a similar or greater degree of self-disclosure.
3. The higher the level of trust, the higher the level of self-disclosure.

Provide Consistency of Experience

1. Enforce consistent restrictions.
2. Provide consistency in attitude.
3. Provide patient with information about the availability of time to spend with him. Meet with patient at agreed-upon time(s).
4. Give patient information about changes in his schedule or surroundings.

Demonstrate Sensitivity to and Respect for Patient

1. Show honesty and moral integrity.
2. Allow for privacy as needed.
3. Create an atmosphere enabling patient to express himself freely.

4. Convey hope, optimism, and expectation for patient's ability to change, grow, and develop a more adaptive behavioral response. Support healthy parts of patient's personality.
5. Explain and provide information to the patient about his condition and the health care setting in which he is being treated in words that he can understand. Use informational booklets and other teaching materials as appropriate.
6. Be aware that the accuracy of one's perceptions of a patient could be influenced by any of the following:
   a. *Assimilation effect*—Viewing a person's opinions more similar to one's own than they are.
   b. *Contrast effect*—Viewing a person's opinions more unlike one's own than they are.
   c. *Primary effect*—Making judgments on first impressions.
   d. *Halo effect*—Tendency to assume that a person possesses positively valued traits if the observer is generally impressed with the person, or the converse.
   e. *Concern with central traits*—Perceiving others on the basis of whether or not they possess traits that one positively values.
   f. *Stereotyping*—Assigning selected traits to a person because he belongs to a certain group.
   g. *Self-defense mechanisms*—Especially if overused.
   h. *Assumed liking*—Assuming that people we like will like us and our preferences, or the converse.
7. Permit expression of negative feelings. Avoid retaliation and punishment for behavior expressed.
8. Focus on strengths and potential of patient.
9. Avoid increasing anxiety unnecessarily.

Express Empathy

1. Perceive and recognize patient's private, inner experiences and feelings.
   a. Use open-ended questions focusing on feelings.
   b. Reflect patient's feelings.
   c. Focus on "being with" patient.
2. Develop awareness of own response to patient.
   a. Recognize interaction of own experiences and those described by patient.
   b. Develop awareness of own response to assist in grasping dynamic meaning, significance, and purpose of patient's experiences and feelings.
   c. Develop sense of meaning for that which patient is not fully aware.
   d. Achieve an ongoing awareness of perceptual, cognitive, and affective aspects of patient.
3. Communicate accurate, sensitive understanding.
   a. Selectively use self-disclosure. Share experiences that model expression of feelings and exploration, as well as help patient recognize that he is not alone.
   b. Communicate understanding of feelings expressed by patient.

c. Communicate understanding of underlying feelings and assumptions implied by patient.
4. Express highest level of empathy possible—at least Level 3. At Levels 4 and 5 even more empathy is expressed. Levels 1 and 2 are not therapeutic and are therefore not described. For Levels 3, 4, and 5, see subsequent items.
   a. Characteristics of Level 3 expression of empathy
      (1) Communicate understanding of patient's feelings at the same level as he expresses them.
      (2) Respond by accurately reflecting patient's state of being.
      (3) Seek to explore meaning of feelings that are expressed in a vague manner.
   b. Characteristics of Level 4 expression of empathy:
      (1) Communicate understanding of underlying feelings of patient, somewhat deeper than actual level expressed.
      (2) Communicate verbally in a manner adding somewhat deeper meaning than that which is verbally expressed by patient.
   c. Characteristics of Level 5 expression of empathy:
      (1) Respond by adding significantly to the meaning and affect that the patient expresses explicitly.
      (2) Communicate accurately the meaning and affect of the patient's deeper feelings.

Demonstrate Unconditional Positive Regard and Acceptance of the Patient in His Uniqueness

1. Communicate value of the patient's being and potential.
   a. Preserve patient's individuality, opinions, uniqueness, and feelings.
   b. Be nonevaluative and nonjudgmental.
   c. Avoid reducing self-esteem of patient.
2. Demonstrate sincere and nonpossessive caring and concern.
3. Communicate openness and willingness to engage in a theapeutic nurse–patient relationship.
4. Convey acceptance of patient's uniqueness, but do not approve inappropriate behavior.
5. Remain objective in observing and identifying reasons for patient's behavior.
6. Make self available.
   a. Do not communicate indifference or rejection.
   b. Offer presence and spend time with patient.
   c. Demonstrate concern, understanding, and interest.
7. Develop and use open-minded, accurate, and flexible interpersonal perceptions.
8. Don't attempt to negate patient's perception of an experience by comments such as, "Oh, it can't be that bad!"
9. Demonstrate availability to patient by taking time to assist him therapeutically.
10. Attempt to understand patient's perspective and feelings.

11. Demonstrate awareness and understanding of differences in cultural and subcultural values and customs.
12. Demonstrate flexibility—that is, a responsiveness to change in conditions.

Use Confrontation Appropriately

1. Communicate to patient growth-defeating discrepancies in his behavior, feelings, perceptions, and thinking.
2. Encourage examination of these discrepancies.
3. Assist patient in becoming fully aware of an aspect of his behavior or problem.
4. While using confrontation, convey a constructive interest, caring, and a high level of respect for patient's ability to grow.
5. Use appropriate timing when using confrontation.
6. Utilize empathy, authenticity, respect, and so on to facilitate self-confrontation. Avoid overuse of nurse-initiated confrontation.

3
Psychiatric Assessment of the Adult

CONCEPTUAL FRAMEWORK FOR PSYCHIATRIC NURSING PRACTICE

See Figure 3-1.
1. Human beings are in continuous interplay with their environment.
2. Human beings possess the potential ability to cope with stressors, meet needs, and attain goals through adaptive strategies, skills, and processes.
3. Adaptive strategies, skills, and processes include the following:
   a. *Interaction*—Exchanging, interchanging, or linking matter, energy, persons, or objects between the person and the environment.
      (1) *Exchanging*—Matter and energy interchange.
      (2) *Communicating*—Information interchange.
      (3) *Relating*—Person or object linkage(s) and interaction.
   b. *Action*—Assigning value, selecting alternatives, and taking action.
      (1) *Valuing*—Assigning value, worth, or meaning.
      (2) *Choosing*—Setting priorities and selecting alternatives.
      (3) *Moving*—Taking action within one's environment.
   c. *Awareness*—Alertness, feeling, knowing/perception.
      (1) *Waking*—Level of alertness.
      (2) *Feeling*—Sensation and mood.
      (3) *Knowing*—Ability to perceive, store, and use information accurately.

The Nursing Process

The nursing process is an interactive, systematic, problem-solving process that is utilized to fulfill the goal of nursing and assist the client to achieve a maximum level of wellness. It should be utilized throughout the one-to-one nurse–patient relationship.

A. Assessment

The systematic and continuous collection of data about the health status of the client.

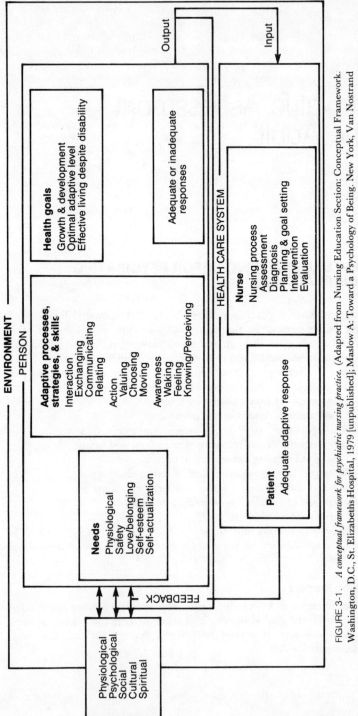

FIGURE 3-1. *A conceptual framework for psychiatric nursing practice.* (Adapted from Nursing Education Section: Conceptual Framework. Washington, D.C., St. Elizabeths Hospital, 1979 [unpublished]; Maslow A: Toward a Psychology of Being. New York, Van Nostrand Rheinhold, 1968; Riehl J and Roy C: Conceptual Models for Nursing Practice. New York, Appleton-Century-Crofts, 1974; Kim M, Moritz D: Classification of Nursing Diagnoses: Proceedings of Third and Fourth National Conference. New York, McGraw-Hill, 1982; Kim M, McFarland G, McLane A (eds): Classification of Nursing Diagnoses: Proceedings of the Fifth National Conference. St Louis, CV Mosby, 1984.)

1. Guidelines for structuring the interview.
   a. Utilize a nursing history guide during the interview to collect data.
   b. Provide for privacy, physical comfort, and freedom from interruption during the interview.
   c. Conduct interview with sensitivity so as to facilitate the beginning of a positive nurse–patient relationship.
   d. Explain the purpose, nature, and length of the interview.
   e. Inform patient that information gained will be utilized to assist in his treatment and shared with appropriate staff.
   f. Ask about the nature of the patient's problem and current life situation.
   g. Observe for both verbal and nonverbal expressions, changes in mood, and difficulties in answering any questions.
   h. Ask questions in a concrete and simple way. Do not delve into complex issues in depth during the first interview.
   i. Utilize a conceptual framework for nursing practice to guide observations, interviewing, and assessment.
   j. Follow health care agency guidelines for charting observations and assessment.
2. *Process recordings*—Written records of the communication of both the nurse and the patient, especially during individual nurse psychotherapy when indicated.
   a. May be used by a nurse expert to review and supervise the one-to-one nurse–patient relationship developed by the nurse or nursing student being supervised.
   b. Can include an analysis of
      (1) The nurse's thoughts, observations, feelings, and interventions (including the treatment goal).
      (2) The patient's responses.
      (3) The total interaction.

B. Nursing diagnosis

Formulated from an analysis of patient assessment and the data collected.

C. Planning

1. Develop behavioral goals after adequate assessment and formulation of the nursing diagnosis.
2. Plan with input from patient, as much as possible.

D. Intervention

1. Intervention strategies should be designed to help patient achieve formulated behavioral goals.
2. A conceptual framework for nursing practice serves to guide planning and design intervention strategies.

E. Evaluation

1. Determine extent to which goals have been met.
2. Data resulting from evaluation are used to plan and redesign intervention strategies to meet goals, to revise goals, or to formulate new goals, as necessary.

Psychiatric Nursing Assessment of the Adult Patient

1. General Information

   Name: _____

   Address: _____

   Phone: _____

   Age: _____

   Sex: _____

   Marital status: _____

   Name of spouse, relative, or friend: _____

   Occupation/Education: _____

   General appearance: _____

   Other: _____

2. Initial Assessment Parameters

   Vital signs: _____

   Allergies: _____

   Neurological status: _____

   　　Level of consciousness: _____

   　　History of seizures: _____

   　　History of blackouts: _____

   Suicidal thoughts/behavior: _____

   Homocidal thoughts/behavior: _____

   Current medications: _____

   Use of street drugs or alcohol: _____

   Weight (loss or gain): _____

   Dentures/dental problems: _____

   Skin condition: _____

   Vision: _____

Psychiatric Nursing Assessment of the Adult Patient (*Continued*)

Hearing: _____

3. Interaction (Exchanging, Communicating, Relating)

DOCUMENT OBSERVATIONS ABOUT SELF-CARE ABILITIES OR LIMITATIONS.

Eating/drinking: _____

Eliminating: _____

Breathing: _____

Circulation: _____

General appearance/grooming/hygiene: _____

Other (specify): _____

Current physical problems: _____

Current treatments and medications: _____

Previous and current use of health care resources: _____

Previous mental or physical illness: _____

General level of growth and development: _____

Communication skills: _____

    With staff: _____

    With spouse: _____

    With children: _____

    With others (specify): _____

Relating: _____

    Ability to trust: _____

    Expression of sexuality: _____

    Self-control: _____

    Manner of expression of needs/goals: _____

    Degree of social interaction: _____

    Style of social interaction: _____

(*Continued*)

Psychiatric Nursing Assessment of the Adult Patient (*Continued*)

Attitude toward perceived current role status: _____

   Social network: _____

   Relationship with spouse and/or significant other(s): _____

Significant others' response to patient's illness: _____

Work history and current status: _____

Recreational activities and hobbies: _____

Arrests, court dates, probation: _____

4. Action (Valuing, Choosing, Moving)

Patient's perception/meaning of current mental illness & cause(s): _____

_____

Beliefs about illness and health and personal health goals: _____

_____

Patient's attitudes/beliefs toward hospitalization and health care

personnel: _____

_____

Patient's expectations and goals for current hospitalization: _____

_____

_____

_____

Past and current compliance with prescribed treatment and health

instructions: _____

_____

Coping skills used: _____

_____

Religion/spiritual beliefs: _____

Decision-making abilities/limitations: _____

Attitudes toward future worth/value of own life: _____

Psychiatric Nursing Assessment of the Adult Patient (*Continued*)

Suicidal thoughts/behaviors: _____

Activity pattern: _____

5. Awareness (Alertness, Feeling, Knowing/Perception)

Orientation to time, place, person: _____

Arousal level: _____

Level of energy: _____

Sleep/rest pattern: _____

Anxiety: _____

Degree and nature of ambivalence: _____

Guilt and source: _____

Type and change of mood or affect: _____

Frequency and types of physical complaints: _____

Patient's adjustment to types, number, and recency of stressors: _____

Type and use of defense mechanisms: _____

Patient's opinion of himself (who he is, self-worth, etc.): _____

Patient's concerns about his physical appearance: _____

Knowledge about present illness (prevention, treatment, self-care

responsibilities): _____

Knowledge about current medications: _____

Unusual beliefs: _____

Unusual sensations and perceptions: _____

6. Discharge planning: _____

Resources: _____

Outpatient appointments: _____

Home visits: _____

THE MENTAL STATUS REVIEW

The mental status review is usually performed by the psychiatrist or psychiatric clinical nurse specialist. Although the mental status examination may have diminished in importance with the advent of the multiaxial evaluation system of the Diagnostic and Statistical Manual of Mental Disorders, or DSM-III (see further on), it is still commonly utilized. However, it serves as only one component of the overall assessment of mental health.

Objective

To assess the mental functioning and present emotional state of the patient.

General Appearance

Observe the following about the patient:
1. Grooming and dress (slovenly, neat, unkempt, overly meticulous, disheveled, inappropriate, unusual).
2. Facial expression (calm, perplexed, stressed, tense, alert, dazed).
3. Physical appearance (noticeable physical deformities, thin, obese, average weight).
4. Posture (normal, rigid, slouching).
5. Eye contact (eyes closed, eyes open, good contact, avoids contact, stares).

Motor Behavior

Observe for unusual bodily movements, such as the following:
1. *Choreiform movements*—Irregular, involuntary actions of muscles of face and extremities.
2. *Waxy flexibility*—Holding body posture that is imposed by another person for a long time.
3. *Hyperkinesia*—Excessive movement; destructive or assaultive activity.
4. *Compulsion*—Unwanted urge to perform repetitive actions.
5. *Automatism*—Not consciously controlled, automatic, undirected motor activity.
6. *Cataplexy*—Temporary loss of muscle tone precipitated by strong emotions.
7. *Catalepsy*—A trancelike state with loss of voluntary motion.
8. *Stereotypy*—Repetitive, persistent motor activity or speech.
9. *Echopraxia*—Repetitive imitation of another person's movements.
10. *Psychomotor retardation*—Decreased, slowed activity.
11. *Catatonic stupor*—Extreme underactivity.
12. *Catatonic excitement*—Extreme overactivity.
13. *Impulsiveness*—Outbursts of activity that are unpredictable and sudden.
14. *Tics and spasms*—Involuntary twitching and jerking of muscles, usually above the shoulders.

Speech

Observe for speech activity, unusual patterns, or unusual use of words, such as the following:
1. *Verbigeration*—Repetitive, meaningless expression of sentences, phrases, or words.

2. *Rhyming*—Interjecting into the conversation regular, recurring, corresponding sounds at the end of phrases or sentences, as in poetry.
3. *Punning*—Interjecting into the conversation the clever and humorous use of a word or words.
4. *Mutism*—No expression of words or lack of communication over a period of time.
5. *Aphasia*—Partial or total loss of the ability to express self through language or the ability to understand the verbal communication of another person.
6. Unusual rate of speech, volume of voice, or intonation and modulation.

Intellectual Functioning

Assess the patient for the following:

A. Orientation
1. Orientation to time
   Ask the patient to name the month, day of the week, and time and to state how long he has been in the hospital.
2. Orientation to place
   Ask the patient: Where are you now located? What is the name of this place? What is the address of this place?
3. Orientation to person
   Does patient know his name? Does patient know who the person conducting the interview is?

B. Memory
1. Memory for remote events—Ask the patient the following:
   a. Date(s) of marriage(s) and divorce(s), if any.
   b. Birthdate(s) of child(ren), if any.
   c. Birthdates of parents.
   d. Name of grade school, high school, and/or college attended.
   e. Type of position and month and year of employment of first job after high school or college graduation.
2. Memory for recent past events—Ask the patient the following:
   a. Where he lived during past 3 months. Whom living with? Where working?
   b. Which types of recreational activities he is involved in.
3. Memory for recent events—Ask the patient the following:
   a. What he ate for breakfast, lunch, and dinner today.
   b. How he spent yesterday and today.
4. Immediate memory and recall
   a. Administer digit span test. Ask patient to repeat three digits in order presented, then backwards. Repeat procedure for 4, 5, and 6 digits.
   b. Other assessment techniques include asking patient the same question several times during the interview to determine whether the same or a different answer is given.
   c. In another technique, instruct patient to count to 28, stop for 45 seconds, instruct him to count from where he left off to 39, stop again for 3

minutes and engage in neutral conversation, then instruct him to count from where he left off to 50.

5. Abnormal memory or symptoms related to impaired memory, such as amnesia, anterograde amnesia, hysterical amnesia, confabulation, déjà vu, hypermnesia, clang association, and retrospective falsification.

C. Level and fund of knowledge

1. To determine fund of knowledge, ask such questions as: What are the names of three countries in Europe? The colors in the American flag? The distance between any two major U.S. cities?
2. Request listing of as many items in different categories, such as U.S. state capitols and fruits.
3. Overall responses to total interview questions are used to assess level of knowledge appropriate on patient's age and socioeconomic, cultural, occupational, and educational background.

D. Ability for calculation

Instruct patient to subtract 7 from 100 and to keep subtracting 7s, allowing up to 30 seconds between calculations.

E. Ability to think abstractly or to make generalizations

1. Ask patient to interpret a proverb particular to his subculture, or
2. Use object sorting test by having patient group toy objects according to use.

Perception

Observe for signs of altered or abnormal awareness of self or environment, such as the following:

1. *Hallucinations*—Sensory perceptions for which there are no external stimuli. These can be visual, olfactory, auditory, tactile, gustatory, or kinesthetic.
2. *Hypnagogic hallucinations*—Misperceptions occurring as patient is falling asleep for which there is no basis in reality.
3. *Hypnopompic hallucinations*—Misperceptions occurring as patient is waking up for which there is no basis in reality.
4. *Illusion*—Misinterpretation of an actual, existing external stimuli by any of the senses.

A. Attitude

Observe for changes in patient's general manner of feeling, thinking, or behavior during the interview as evidenced by his being any one or more of the following: cooperative, outgoing, withdrawn, evasive, sarcastic, aggressive, perplexed, hostile, arrogant, dramatic, ingratiating, submissive, fearful, seductive, uncooperative, impatient, remote, resistant, unfeeling, apprehensive, or apathetic.

Affective State

Observe for unusual mood or expression of emotions, such as the following:

1. *Euphoria*—Excessive feeling of emotional and physical well-being inappropriate for actual environmental stimuli.

2. *Flat affect*—Less than normal expression of feelings.
3. *Blunting*—Loss of affective capacity.
4. *Elation*—High degree of confidence, boastfulness, uncritical optimism, and joy accompanied by increased motor activity.
5. *Exultation*—Affective reaction extending beyond elation and accompanied by feelings of grandeur.
6. *Ecstasy*—Overpowering feeling of joy and rapture.
7. *Anxiety*—Apprehensive, uneasy, and worried feeling usually of unconscious, intrapsychic origin.
8. *Fear*—Apprehensive, uneasy, and worried feeling related to a known source of danger, usually externally based.
9. *Ambivalence*—Expression of the existence of two opposing feelings or emotions at the same time.
10. *Depersonalization*—One's feeling that he or his environment is unreal.
11. *Irritability*—Feeling characterized by impatience, annoyance, and easy provocation to anger.
12. *Rage*—Furious, uncontrolled anger.
13. *Lability*—Quick change of expression of mood or feelings.
14. *Depression*—Feeling characterized by sadness, dejection, and gloom.

Thought Processes and Content

Observe for the following:

1. *Blocking*—Sudden cessation of flow of thinking and speech related to strong emotions.
2. *Flight of ideas*—Rapid conversation with logically unconnected shifting of topics.
3. *Word salad*—Combination of phrases, words, and sentences that are disconnected and incoherent.
4. *Perseveration*—Pathological repetition of a sentence, phrase, or word.
5. *Neologisms*—Use of new expressions, phrases, or words or creation of a new meaning for accepted expressions, phrases, or words.
6. *Circumstantiality*—Interjection of great detail and incidental material that have no primary significance to the central idea of the conversation.
7. *Echolalia*—Repetitive imitation of another person's speech.
8. *Condensation*—Process of reducing several ideas into one symbol.
9. *Delusion*—False belief kept despite nonsupportive evidence.
10. *Phobia*—Strong, persistent, abnormal fear of an object or situation.
11. *Obsession*—Persistent, unwanted, recurring thought.
12. *Hypochondriasis*—Morbid concern for one's health and feeling ill without any actual medical basis.

Judgment

Observe patient's ability to problem solve and choose among alternatives based on reality.

Alertness

Observe patient for levels of alertness (drowsiness, hyperalertness, somnolence, intermittent alertness and drowsiness, stupor).

THE MULTIAXIAL EVALUATION SYSTEM OF THE DIAGNOSTIC AND STATISTICAL MANUAL OF MENTAL DISORDERS (DSM-III)

1. The Diagnostic and Statistical Manual of Mental Disorders (DSM-III) "is a methodical attempt to define, in terms of descriptive psychopathology, the wide range of mental disorders currently encountered in clinical practice."[1]
2. The DMS-III recommends the evaluation of a patient's psychological and physical functioning, stressors contributing to the development of a psychological disorder, and strengths and limitations.
3. In using the DSM-III, the clinician takes into consideration prior history of illness and family history and looks at specific behaviors more specifically. In order to arrive at a differential diagnoses, the clinician views the patient both longitudinally and cross-sectionally.
4. The five axes in the DSM-III on which the patient is evaluated are as follows:[2]
   a. Axis I—Clinical syndromes:
      (1) Conditions not attributable to a mental disorder that are a focus of attention or treatment
      (2) Additional codes
   b. Axis II—Personality disorders; specific developmental disorders.
   c. Axis III—Physical disorders and conditions.
   d. Axis IV—Severity of psychosocial stressors.
   e. Axis V—Highest level of adaptive functioning during past year.

PSYCHOLOGICAL TESTING

Intelligence Testing

To assess cognitive and intellectual abilities, usually administered by a psychologist.

> *Wechsler Adult Intelligence Scale (WAIS)*—Most widely used standardized test of general intelligence.

Personality Testing

To assess personality functioning and psychodynamics, usually administered by a psychologist.

1. *Thematic Apperception Test (TAT)*—A projective test consisting of a series of 30 pictures. A number of these are presented to the patient with instructions that a story be constructed or created about the picture.
2. *Rorschach Test*—A projective test consisting of a set of 10 inkblots. The patient is asked what he sees in the inkblot, what it looks like, and what it suggests.
3. *Draw a Person Test (DAP)*—The patient is asked to draw one or more persons and possibly a house, a tree, the family, or an animal. The clinician may also question the patient about the drawing. It is a projective test used for personality analysis and in screening for organic brain damage.
4. *Bender-Gestalt Test*—The patient is presented with nine cards, one at a time,

and is asked to copy the geometric designs on them. The test is used to detect organic pathology and is also employed as a projective technique to assess personality functioning.

5. *Sentence Completion Test (SCT)*—The patient is presented with 75 to 100 sentence stems that he is asked to complete with the first response that comes into mind. The test taps much conscious data and can identify the patient's preoccupations, concerns, fears, and goals.

6. *Minnesota Multiphasic Personality Inventory (MMPI)*—A 500-item questionnaire designed to measure major aspects of personality related to hypomania, paranoia, hypochondriasis, hysteria, psychopathic deviation, psychasthenia, schizophrenia, masculinity/femininity, and depression.

REFERENCES

1. Skodol A, Spitzer R, Williams J: Teaching and learning DSM-III. Am J Psychiatry 138 (12): 1582, 1981
2. Diagnostic and Statistical Manual of Mental Disorders, 3rd ed, p 23, Washington DC, The American Psychiatric Association, 1980

4
Nursing Diagnoses in Caring for the Psychiatric Patient

The nursing diagnoses selected for discussion in this chapter relate primarily to the care of the individual psychiatric patient. However, these nursing diagnoses can be applied to other patients whose nursing care is enhanced by the appropriate diagnoses and by the planning and implementation of psychosocial interventions.

The majority of nursing diagnoses outlined in this chapter are selected from the approved list of the North American Nursing Diagnoses Association (NANDA). A few labels have been modified, and some have been added as a result of ongoing clinical observation, colleague input, research, and literature review. For example, the authors use the nursing diagnosis label "communication, impaired" instead of the label on the NANDA list, "communication, impaired verbal." (See research on impaired communication by McFarland and Naschinski, 1985.[1])

Other nursing diagnoses labels (*e.g.*, depressive behavior) have been added because there are gaps in the current NANDA list as developed for the nursing care of psychiatric clients. Noteworthy is the fact that Carpenito (1984)[2] identified the nursing diagnosis label: "ineffective individual coping related to depression in response to identified stressors." Whatever the eventual outcome in terms of the actual label accepted for this phenomenon, it must be understood that NANDAs work is developmental and ongoing. The fact that the classification system as currently developed has "large gaps in the structure at all levels, that is, unnamed phenomena or categories of phenomena" was supported by the work of Kritek and her group at the 5th National Conference on the Classification of Nursing Diagnoses (Kim et al., 1984).[3] As nursing diagnostic labels are developed, utilized, and tested in clinical practice, it is important that input be provided to NANDAs ongoing developmental work.

Definition and Characteristics of Nursing Diagnoses

1. *Nursing diagnosis* is a word or phrase summarizing a set of empirical indicators—defining characteristics—linked to contributing factors or etiology, when possible, and representing actual or potential altered patterns of human functioning, which nurses are licensed to treat.[4]

2. Nursing diagnoses approved by the North American Nursing Diagnoses Association (NANDA) are as follows[5]:

> Activity intolerance
>
> Activity intolerance, potential
>
> Airway clearance, ineffective
>
> Anxiety
>
> Bowel elimination, alteration in: constipation
>
> Bowel elimination, alteration in: diarrhea
>
> Bowel elimination, alteration in: incontinence
>
> Breathing pattern, ineffective
>
> Cardiac output, alteration in: decreased
>
> Comfort, alteration in: pain
>
> Communication, impaired: verbal
>
> Coping, family: potential for growth
>
> Coping, ineffective family: compromised
>
> Coping, ineffective family: disabling
>
> Coping, ineffective individual
>
> Diversional activity, deficit
>
> Family process, alteration in
>
> Fear
>
> Fluid volume, alteration in: excess
>
> Fluid volume deficit, actual (1)
>
> Fluid volume deficit, actual (2)
>
> Fluid volume deficit, potential
>
> Gas exchange, impaired
>
> Grieving, anticipatory
>
> Grieving, dysfunctional
>
> Health maintenance, alteration in
>
> Home maintenance management, impaired
>
> Injury, potential for
>
> Knowledge deficit (specify)
>
> Mobility, impaired physical
>
> Noncompliance (specify)
>
> Nutrition, alteration in: less than body requirements

Nutrition, alteration in: more than body requirements

Nutrition, alteration in: potential for more than body requirements

Oral mucous membrane, alteration in

Parenting, alteration in: actual or potential

Powerlessness

Rape trauma syndrome

Self-care deficit: feeding, bathing/hygiene, dressing/grooming, toileting

Self-concept, disturbance in: body image, self-esteem, role performance, personal identity

Sensory-perceptual alteration: visual, auditory, kinesthetic, gustatory, tactile, olfactory

Sexual dysfunction

Skin integrity, impairment of: actual

Skin integrity, impairment of: potential

Sleep pattern disturbance

Social isolation

Spiritual distress

Thought processes, alteration in

Tissue perfusion, alteration in: cerebral, cardiopulmonary, renal, gastrointestinal, peripheral

Urinary elimination, alteration in patterns

Violence, potential for: self-directed or directed at others

Framework for Discussing Nursing Diagnoses

1. *Definition*—A brief description of the diagnostic label.
2. *General principles*—Relevant principles discussed when appropriate.
3. *Etiology*—The contributing factor(s) or cause(s).
4. *Defining characteristics*—Includes the empirical indicators or behavioral manifestations. Key concepts or etiological factors will be discussed for some diagnoses.
5. *Nursing assessment*—Initial or ongoing diagnosis-specific assessment factors supplemental to the overall assessment parameters outlined in Chapter 3. The questions and statements listed serve as guidelines for assessment and should be adapted as necessary.
6. *Goals and Nursing Interventions*—Includes goals followed by nursing interventions designed to achieve each specific goal.
   a. In designing an individual patient care plan, the nurse can restate goals in patient behavioral outcome terms, if desired.
   b. The nurse selects interventions from among those listed to individualize the nursing care plan for a specific patient.
7. *Health education and prevention*—Diagnostics-specific content useful in patient teaching or as preventive measures.

8. *Evaluation*—Outcome criteria will be specified.
9. There are differences in the conceptual level of abstraction of the listed diagnoses. The best diagnosis(es) for a patient should be determined on the basis of an analysis of the available assessment data collected.
10. Nursing diagnosis can be changed as more data, warranting the change, become available.
11. The established nursing diagnosis(es) for a patient gives direction to the next phases of the nursing process—planning, intervention, and evaluation.
   a. The etiological or contributing factor(s) should be identified, if possible, and added to the main phrase of the nursing diagnosis.
   b. The two parts are linked with the words "related to."
      This is done to clarify documentation of the relationships of the components of the nursing conceptual framework, which, in turn, affects nursing care planning and intervention.

AGGRESSION, INAPPROPRIATE

Definition
1. *Inappropriate aggression*—A forceful, inappropriate, nonadaptive verbal or physical action that may result from such feelings/emotional states as anger, anxiety, tension, guilt, and hostility, in turn resulting from a variety of precipitating factors.
2. *Violence*—Pursuit of own interests by force; at extreme end of aggression continuum.

General Principles
1. Inappropriate aggression may be
   a. learned and perpetuated by motives, attitudes, and rationalizations supported by subculture;
   b. produced or perpetuated by hospital social structure (*e.g.*, coercion, regimentation, personal space invasion).
2. See Table 4-1, Model of Aggression.

Etiology
1. Fear
2. Guilt
3. Anxiety
4. Anger
5. Repressed resentment
6. Grief
7. Powerlessness
8. Thwarted goals
9. Thwarted needs
10. Threatened goal progression
11. Threat to physiological need satisfaction
12. Threat to security need satisfaction
13. Threat to belonging need satisfaction
14. Threatened self-concept

TABLE 4-1. **Model of Aggression**

Possible Causes	Possible Resulting Feelings	Possible Resulting Responses
Frustration		*Adaptive Response*
Loss of dignity		Use of coping skills and strategies result-
Fear		ing in resolution, including constructive
Need to test reality	Anxiety	expression of aggression as in problem-solving or realistic defense.
Physical impairment (*e.g.*, minimal brain dysfunction)	Guilt	OR
Inferiority and low self-esteem	Tension	*Inadequate Adaptive Response—Inappropriate Expression of Aggression*
Repressed resentment, hate, or hostility	Anger	Defensive actions—designed to meet personal needs, achieve goals and protect
Grief (anger phase)	Hostility	self including both inappropriate verbal or physical expression of aggression.
Perceived threat		Offensive actions—designed to punish or
Threat of intimacy		destroy including verbal hostility, physical assault, or violence.
Perceptual or cognitive distortion		Direct action against cause—includes
Social milieu (*e.g.*, rejection from significant others or subculture expression of aggression)		other or self-directed physical or verbal aggression.
Helplessness		Indirect action against cause—includes scape-goating; acting-out; overuse of
Thwarting of goals as career progression		displacement, projection, introjection, reaction-formation, or somatization; or
Thwarting of needs for power, control, authority, attention		passive-aggressive behavior, such as gossiping, round-about derogation, derogatory jokes, slamming doors, temper
Ward milieu (*e.g.*, staff conflict, over-crowding, *etc.*)		tantrums, negativism, resentment, irritability or postponements.

15. Loss of dignity
16. Subculture milieu
17. Rejection by significant other
18. Staff conflict
19. Physical disorder
20. Substance abuse disorder

Defining Characteristics

1. Inappropriate forceful goal-directed verbal action
2. Inappropriate forceful goal-directed physical action
3. Passive aggressive behavior

4. Slamming doors
5. Derogatory jokes
6. Gossiping
7. Round-about derogation
8. Acting-out
9. Scapegoating
10. Negativism
11. Irritability
12. Temper tantrums
13. Resentment
14. Overuse of mental mechanisms
15. Verbal hostility
16. Cursing
17. Screaming/shouting
18. Inappropriate defensive verbalizations
19. Intimidation
20. Damaging inanimate objects
21. Physical assault of animals
22. Physical assault/injury of persons
23. Inappropriate physical defensive action
24. Destructive offensive actions
25. Self-inflicted physical harm

Nursing Assessment
1. What is the nature of the patient's aggressive behavior? Preceding events? Precipitants? Place of occurrence? Actual behavior, including intensity, target, degree of inner controls?
2. What is the patient's perception of self, environment?
3. What is the meaning behind the aggressive behavior?
4. Determine patient's prior methods of coping with stress-producing situations and ways used to gain self-control.
5. How does the patient cope with anger?
   a. Internalizes, becomes depressed?
   b. Unable to identify source, displacement?
   c. Able to identify source but unable to express directly? Passive aggressive?
   d. Identifies source along with direct and appropriate or inappropriate expression?
6. Assess potential for violent behavior by considering factors such as
   a. Past history of arrests and violent behavior
   b. History of life stressors resulting in bitterness
   c. Unstable family situation characterized by quarreling
   d. Violence displayed by significant others, especially parental brutality
   e. High interest in, and availability of, weapons
   f. Low self-esteem without involvement in constructive activities
   g. Toxic state from alcohol or drug abuse
   h. Presence of persecutional delusions
   i. History of physical impairment, such as minimal brain dysfunction

   j. Organization and rehearsal of plans for violent act

   k. Absence of reliable significant other(s)

   l. Degree of reversibility of predisposing conditions

   m. Methods of dealing with similar past situations

7. Continue observations for
   a. Behavioral changes indicating increasing anxiety, guilt, anger
   b. Homicidal or suicidal ideation
   c. Inappropriate aggression
      (1) What were the preceding events, including ward milieu?
      (2) What were the precipitating factors?
      (3) What actually happened?
      (4) How does the patient perceive the event?
   d. Ward milieu, including staff ability to cope effectively with own emotions
   e. Possession of any weapons
   f. Change in ability to resolve anxiety, anger, tension, or guilt in an acceptable way
   g. Other acts of aggression on ward that seem unrelated

Goals and Nursing Interventions

A. To reduce/eliminate inappropriate aggression and identify and express feelings.

1. Assist patient in dealing with anger.
   a. Provide feedback on nonverbal behavior to help patient identify anger.
   b. Develop relationship in which patient can be angry and can learn to distinguish between feelings and actions.
   c. Have patient practice verbalizing angry feelings in a minimally threatening situation.
   d. Assist in identifying sources of anger.
   e. Explore and aid in developing alternate methods of expressing anger, including using the direct approach.
2. Reduce passive-aggressive behavior.
   a. Observe and document behavior.
   b. After having developed positive relationship with patient, confront him, pointing out behaviors and their consequences.
   c. Set limits and give positive reinforcement for appropriate behavior.
3. Develop therapeutic ward milieu.
   a. Provide opportunity through group meetings for staff and patients to discuss reactions and feelings about inappropriate aggression and to resolve patient–staff conflict.
   b. Resolve conflict.
   c. Work through phases of planned change.
4. Mutually develop goals with patient for more appropriate expression of anger, hostility, anxiety, tension, or guilt. Seek alternatives that can be used after discharge.
5. Analyze own perceptions of patient. Avoid stereotyping or "expecting" physical aggression.

6. Assist patient in reducing cognitive distortion and developing alternative perspective about himself and the causes of his aggression.
7. Help reduce anxiety.
8. Point out consequences of inappropriate aggression.
9. Prevent suicide or homicide.
10. Evaluate need for group or family therapy.
11. Provide outlets for feelings engendered (*e.g.*, activity groups, punching bags, clay, sports, art, music).
12. Help patient recognize cause and effect among cause, emotions, and aggressive behavior displayed.
13. Develop behavior-modification approaches for selected aggressive behaviors.
14. Explore patient's past experiences with aggressive behavior and what rewards his current aggressive behavior achieves for him.
15. Provide peer role models who demonstrate more adaptive behavioral responses.

B. To lessen risk or prevent injury to self and others and recognize potential for inappropriate aggression.

1. If patient possesses a weapon
   a. Don't attempt to grab it, unless there are enough staff members present.
   b. Request that weapon be deposited in a neutral place.
   c. If threatened with weapon, place protective barrier between self and weapon, such as mattress or chair.
2. Suport ego.
   a. Use honest, empathic, firm approach.
   b. Avoid accusatory approach and increasing guilt.
3. Recognize potential for inappropriate aggression and intervene prior to expression.
4. Be cautious and avoid facade of bravado. Do convey security and don't exhibit fear or panic.
5. Provide opportunity for verbalization of feelings, especially anger: Attempt to "talk down."
6. Do not be hasty in attempts to uncover precipitants, but acknowledge patient's tension. State desire to help patient regain control.
7. Set consistent limits on type and degree of inappropriate aggression that is tolerated.
8. Pose well-timed questions about what the patient may be experiencing.
9. Be aware of potentially stressful situations for patients, and document and communicate any change in behavior.
10. If physical aggression is imminent or occurring, approach patient quietly with staff and, if indicated, use a well-planned method of physical restraint.
11. Do not ignore threats of physical aggression.
12. Be available to patient during periods of increasing tension.
13. Respect patient's need for personal space.
14. Provide consistent set of expectations for patient to develop self-control.

15. Explore options for more constructive outlets for inappropriate aggression.
16. Be as truthful as possible.
17. Remove external object that patient fears, if possible.
18. Recognize need for clearcut staff–patient boundaries.
19. When therapist is verbally threatened
    a. Continue patient contact.
    b. Explore precipitants of threat.
    c. Permit verbalizations of feelings associated with threat.
    d. Assist patient in realizing link between cause, subsequent feelings, and verbal threat.
20. When verbal and nonverbal cues indicate physical aggression
    a. Do not avoid but interact early with patient.
    b. Convey acceptance of person but not of physical aggression.
    c. Avoid retaliatory behaviors.
    d. Permit verbalization of feelings.
    e. Suggest constructive physical outlets, such as use of punching bag.
    f. Suggest use of a quiet area until self-control is fully regained.
21. Maintain stable, therapeutic ward milieu for brain-damaged patients.
22. Develop and implement well-planned, orderly method of restraint for violent patient.
23. Be aware of potential target for patient's physical aggressions.
24. Determine and anticipate need for medications, physical restraints, seclusion, or mechanical restraints, and utilize, following physician's protocol or requests.
25. Ask patient whether medications are desired and encourage patient to take them to prevent further agitation.
26. If medications are refused, offer them again a short time later.
27. If agitated, administer medications after patient has been physically restrained in flat position.
28. Discuss violence and physical aggression with patient after the episode.
29. Communicate that staff members are attempting to solve the immediate problem.
30. Avoid sudden movements with a violent patient.
31. To avoid violence
    a. Observe, plan, and act.
    b. Give one staff member final authority on method of restraint to be used.
    c. Give staff specific instructions.
    d. Use institutional policy as guideline.
    e. Have more staff present than needed to communicate strength.
    f. Do not use force.
    g. Use pillows, mattress, or chair to ward off blows.
    h. Remove other patients from potentially dangerous area.
32. Use self-protective devices to deal with actual physical aggression: Do not inflict pain or injury.
    a. Controlled breathing—Inhale and exhale deeply and sharply before physical action to protect self.

    b. Movement—Move while speaking to agitated patient so he can't predict exact location.

    c. Stance—Place feet shoulder-width apart, forward foot in front, and back foot at 90° angle from forward foot.

    d. Utilize protective fall.

    e. Observation—Observe patient's eyes because he will observe body part that will be attacked.

    f. Protective actions

      (1) Deflect patient action by self-defense techniques.

      (2) Use counterpressure.

      (3) Use body pressure points.

      (4) Seek assistance as soon as possible.

Health Education and Prevention

1. To prevent inappropriate aggression, teach patient to

    a. Recognize warning signs, symptoms, and feelings preceding occurrence.

    b. Avoid toxic substances, such as alcohol, which can impair judgment.

    c. Practice self-control and appropriate expression of feelings and aggression beginning with precipitants evoking minor tension, anger, guilt, or anxiety.

    d. Seek psychiatric assistance when he feels need for help in establishing self-control.

2. List phone numbers of hot line and professionals who can be contacted when need arises.

3. Use relaxation techniques.

Evaluation/Outcome Criteria

1. Aggression expressed appropriately by patient:

    a. Problem-solving

    b. Engaging in realistic and constructive self-defense

    c. Respecting the personal integrity of others

    d. Utilizing assertive communication skills

ANXIETY: MILD, MODERATE, SEVERE, EXTREME (PANIC)

Definition

1. *Anxiety*—An uncomfortable warning of varying intensity of an impending subjective danger for which the source of danger is unknown.

2. *Normal anxiety*—Does not involve repressive or other defensive mechanisms.

3. *Neurotic anxiety*—Involves repression and other defensive mechanisms.

General Principles

1. Anxiety can be experienced at conscious, preconscious, or unconscious levels.

2. Response to anxiety can be constructive (task-oriented behavior) or destructive (defensive-oriented reactions).

3. When the anxiety level exceeds person's adaptive coping strategies, mal-adaptive patterns of behavior may result.
4. The same stressor will not lead to anxiety or to the same level of anxiety in all persons.
5. Anxiety can manifest itself in phobic disorders, anxiety states, or other maladaptive behaviors.

Etiology

1. Threat to self concept
2. Threat to personal security system
3. Threat to value system ideals, or beliefs
4. Interpersonal transmission and contagion
5. Maturational or situational crises
6. Threat to meaningful interpersonal relationships and patterns
7. Threat to stable environment
8. Threat to, or change in, role functioning
9. Perceived or actual change in socioeconomic status
10. Threat to, or change in, health status
11. Unconscious conflict
12. Terminal illness or threat of death
13. Adverse interpersonal relationships, especially in childhood
14. Perceived or actual failure of adaptive coping skills
15. Unmet needs
16. Perceived or actual threat to goal achievement

Defining Characteristics

A. Mild anxiety

1. Slight discomfort
2. Enhanced ability to deal with stressor
3. Increased awareness, problem-solving abilities, perceptual field, and alertness as well as the ability to see more connections between events
4. Sleeplessness
5. Curiosity, repetitive questioning
6. Constant attention-seeking, belittling
7. Misunderstandings, idle hostility, restlessness, irritability
8. Increased attention on problem situation

B. Moderate anxiety

1. Moderate discomfort
2. Increased ability to concentrate and focus attention on problem situation, concentrate on sensory data relevant to problem, and verbalize; more alert
3. Narrowing of perceptual field, selective inattention, some ability to perceive and understand connections between events
4. Voice tremors, change in voice pitch
5. Increased respiratory rate, heart rate, and muscle tension
6. Shakiness

C. Severe anxiety

1. Tendency to dissociate anxious feelings from self; denial of existence of uncomfortable feelings to protect self
2. Greatly reduced range of perception; focus on small or scattered detail; inability to see connections between events or details
3. Selective inattention; interference with effective functioning
4. Difficult and inappropriate verbalizations; inability to concentrate; purposeless activity; inability to learn
5. Sense of impending doom
6. Hyperventilation; tachycardia; frequency and urgency
7. Nausea, headache, and dizziness

D. Extreme anxiety (panic)

1. Extreme discomfort
2. Unrealistic perception of situation
3. Distortion and enlargement of detail, disruption of perceptual field
4. Inability to speak; unintelligible communication
5. Vomiting; feeling of personality disintegration; immobility

Nursing Assessment

1. Determine level of anxiety manifested by patient.
2. Observe adaptive or maladaptive behavioral responses to anxiety.
3. Observe for stressors or threats to any of the following:
   a. Value system, ideals, and beliefs.
   b. Core or essence of personality.
   c. Self-concept.
   d. Personal security system.
   e. Meaningful interpersonal relationships.
   f. Stability of environment.
   g. Role functioning.
4. Assess ward milieu or interpersonal level of anxiety surrounding patient.
5. Determine behavioral changes or physiological changes indicating anxiety.
6. Determine level of anxiety. Indicate physiological and/or psychological signs and symptoms.
7. Determine what patient has done in past to reduce anxiety.
8. Identify patient's current adaptive and maladaptive strategies for coping with anxiety.
9. Determine resources and strengths available for patient to cope with anxiety.

Goals and Nursing Interventions

A. To reduce anxiety to a level at which problem-solving can be effective.

1. Be a good listener.
2. Engage in recreational and diversional activities aimed at reducing anxiety: group singing, volley ball, ping-pong, walking, swimming, simple

concrete tasks, simple games, routine tasks, housekeeping chores, grooming, puzzles, cards, and so on.

Identify constructive ways patient has reduced anxiety in the past.

3. Develop a positive interpersonal relationship with patient.
4. Administer tranquilizers or sedative drugs as prescribed.
5. Encourage ventilation of feelings, considering readiness of patient.
6. Do not probe.
7. Be calm.
   a. Avoid becoming anxious reciprocally.
   b. Recognize anxiety in self and develop control over own responses.
8. Use short, simple sentences and a calm, firm tone in speaking with a highly anxious patient.
9. Provide simple, brief, and clear information about experiences to be encountered while patient is hospitalized.

   Provide, clarify, or validate information as necessary.
10. Avoid requests for decision-making, asking for cause of behavior, or making interpretations when patient is highly anxious.
11. Convey empathy, unconditional positive regard, and congruence.
12. Offer reassurance, including use of nonverbal behavior such as quiet physical presence and use of touch.
13. Intervene early to prevent escalation of anxiety to severe or extreme levels.
14. Keep highly anxious patient in a calm milieu: Remove patient from stress until he is less sensitive to situation if anxiety level is high.
15. Limit contact with other anxious patients.
16. Convey matter-of-fact attitude that problem is not catastrophic and that a constructive resolution can be found.
17. Avoid anxiety-provoking situations: threats, insincerity, focus on weakness, indiscriminate use of psychiatric or medical terminology, unreasonable demands, indiscriminate use of confrontation of behavior, indifference or unconcerned attitude, interference with patient's rights or goals, judgmental attitude, impatience, and so forth.
18. Mutually develop daily schedule of activities, incorporating patient's preferences and strengths.
19. During short-term hospitalization offer additional support and assistance to patient in dealing with anxiety on admission, on about the fifth day, and upon notification of discharge.
20. Permit crying.
21. Reduce guilt by resolving psychodynamics involved.

B. To recognize presence of anxiety, develop insight into cause and develop adaptive coping strategies and behavioral responses.

1. If anxiety is at low or moderate level
   a. Help patient identify his anxiety by asking questions such as, "Are you uncomfortable right now?" Point out your awareness of his discomfort by providing feedback on nonverbal behaviors that indicate anxiety.
   b. Assist patient in discovering similarity of the immediate situation and

past experiences in which comparable discomfort was experienced. Ask questions such as, "Have you, in the past, ever felt like you feel right now? What was happening then to you? What did you do to feel less anxious?"

c. Ask patient to describe what was desired, thought, or expected before becoming anxious and to discover the relationship of his state of anxiety to consequent adaptive or maladaptive behavior.

d. Explore possible reasons for anxiety with patient: Help patient clarify nature of problem realistically.

e. Assist patient in developing alternative solutions and methods to reduce anxiety; choose solutions for use and encourage trying out solutions.

f. Evaluate results with patient. Encourage task-oriented versus self-oriented evaluation. Seek additional information and alternative action if plan was unsuccessful.

2. Encourage new interests and hobbies.
3. After anxiety is lowered and relationship with staff member is established
   a. Encourage social activities even if patient demonstrates reluctance and fears.
   b. Accompany patient first few times to activity and permit him to leave if he becomes too anxious.
   c. Gradually encourage patient's attendance independent of staff support.
4. Utilize and assist patient in choosing objective environmental interventions to deal with anxiety if he is basically optimistic, open to experience, and flexible.
5. Assist patient in developing a more optimistic and constructive world view if his subjective world is deadened, closed, or distorted. Assist him in reducing life-style of negative expectations.
6. Allow patient freedom to work at his own level and pace in solving his problems.
7. Reduce secondary gains patient achieves from maladaptive behavioral responses.

Health Education and Prevention

1. Explore upcoming events. Use role play to help patient cope with anxiety-provoking encounters.
2. Teach patient
   a. That some anxiety is part of living and that enduring mild and moderate anxiety can enhance learning, problem solving, and movement towards self-actualization.
   b. To observe what is happening, describe it, analyze what he expected and how it differs from the actual situation, develop alternatives to solve problem or change expectations, and validate situation with others.
   c. Assertive communication skills.
   d. Progressive muscular relaxation.
3. Instruct patient to reduce severe or extreme anxiety by talking to someone;

walking; taking part in simple games; performing simple, concrete tasks; participating in sports; or, if anxiety is extreme, seeking professional help.

Evaluation/Outcome Criteria

1. Anxiety reduced or resolved: Reduction or absence in patient of defining characteristics of anxiety, especially extreme or severe levels.
2. Anxiety identified and analyzed; constructive strategies utilized.
   a. Patient identifies presence of anxiety in self.
   b. Patient indicates beginning understanding of cause of anxiety.
   c. Patient utilizes constructive anxiety-reducing strategies.
3. Constructive aspects of anxiety identified: Patient recognizes growth potential of mild or moderate anxiety.

COMMUNICATION, IMPAIRED

Definition

1. *Communication*—A dynamic reciprocal process involving a sender, message, and receiver in which information is exchanged.
2. *Impaired communication*—A communication pattern in which the receiver often arrives at a meaning that differs from that intended by the sender.

General Principles

A. Impaired communication responses include the following:

1. *Impervious response*—Outright failure to acknowledge another's attempt to communicate, suggesting that the speaker is unimportant and does not merit attention (*e.g.*, irrelevant response, no response, interrupting).
2. *Tangential response*—Response that is only to an incidental part of speaker's communication (*e.g.*, shifting focus, responding with "yes" or "no," then talking about something else).
3. *Ambiguous response*—Response that is meaningless because more than one, often conflicting, message is contained (*e.g.*, straddling the fence by saying both "yes" and "no," use of nonverbal communication that is incongruous with verbal communication.
4. *Inadequate response*—Response that is meaningless because the message is lost in trivia, is incomplete, or is overqualified.
5. *Projective response*—A mystifying response in which the speaker implies that he knows what is going on inside the other person or is qualified to judge the correctness of the other's feelings.
6. *Crossed transaction*—The response received is not appropriate, is unexpected, and does not follow the natural order of healthy human interactions as opposed to complimentary transactions.
7. *Ulterior transaction*—The transaction occurs at two levels simultaneously: the social and the psychological.

B. Impaired communication patterns include the following:

1. *Games*—A well-structured series of ulterior transactions leading to a well-defined, predictable, but often painful outcome.

2. *Symmetrical escalation*—One person seeks to make the other conform to expectations that are met with defiance.
3. *Rigid complementarity*—One person is strong and overprotective of the other.

Etiology

1. Emotional state
2. Physical condition(s)
3. Mechanical impairment
4. Developmental related stage
5. Inadequate self-concept
6. Cultural differences
7. Poor communication skills
8. Severe stress(es)

Defining Characteristics

1. Inconsistent verbal and nonverbal messages
2. Inconsistent nonverbal messages
3. Message that is inappropriate for context
4. Inappropriately timed messages
5. Verbosity
6. Laconism
7. Absence of gratification
8. Inability to speak dominant language
9. Reluctance or inability to speak
10. Disorientation
11. Inappropriate selection of words
12. Disparity of punctuation
13. Inadequate listening skills
14. Withdrawal from interaction
15. Inappropriate feedback
16. Speech impediments
17. Reluctance or inability to express feelings

Nursing Assessment

1. Carefully note patient's communication abilities and limitations during the interview.
2. Determine the patient's perceptions about his ability to communicate with others.
3. Find out whether patient has a network of significant others.
4. Determine the perceptions of significant others regarding patient's ability to communicate.
5. Observe for dysfunctional communication responses, such as impervious, tangential, ambiguous, inadequate, and projective responses in patient's interactions.
6. Observe for frequency of crossed transactions, of ulterior transactions, and of type of games in which patient involves himself.

7. Observe for defining characteristics indicative of impaired communication.

Goals and Nursing Interventions

A. To resolve impaired communication

1. Involve patient in transactional analysis group or program in which understanding of transactions and games can be increased.
2. Describe and encourage patient to use active listening skills.
3. Ask patient to examine the effect of communication skills and patterns. Suggest to patient that he request honest feedback on his effect on others.
4. Help patient develop insight into dynamics of relationships.
5. Support use of assertive communication skills.
6. Increase patient's acceptance of positive and negative feedback.
7. Increase patient's awareness of areas in which he can be hurt and of what he is willing to share with others.
8. Teach and support patient's use of communication techniques.
9. Increase patient's awareness of the feelings of others.
10. Reduce patient's need to be overprotective in a relationship.
11. Reduce patient's need to attempt to make others conform to his expectations.
    Teach patient to accept the right of others to have their own attitudes.
12. Help patient develop honest, open way of getting needs met.
13. Assist patient in increasing self-esteem.
14. Help patient increase awareness of strengths and limitations in communicating with others.
15. Encourage increased participation in groups.
16. Help patient develop the ability to give and receive in a relationship.
17. Encourage patient to practice reducing use of dysfunctional communication responses.
    Encourage increased use of assertive communication skills.
18. Help patient tolerate disagreement and resolve conflict.
19. Reduce nagging.
20. Encourage initiation of interactions and communication.
21. Decrease use of generalizations.
22. Point out discrepancies in message and the metacommunication sent.
23. Point out discrepancies in the message sent and the context within which it is sent.
24. Use role playing to practice improved communication skills and techniques.
25. Encourage patient to seek assistance in correcting, modifying, or preventing physical conditions that interfere with communication.
26. Assist in identifying and focusing on relevant stimuli.
27. Assist in modifying or increasing language skills.
28. Reduce faulty perceptions.

Health Education

Teach patient to
1. Request feedback from the other person to make certain that communications are accurately understood; for example,
   "By telling me . . . do you mean . . . ?"
2. Let other person know through feedback what he has overtly or covertly said or the feelings that he has conveyed; for example,
   "You're telling me that the whole experience makes you 'livid'."
3. Respond to other person in a manner that conveys a sincere effort to understand how that person perceives his world; for example,
   "As you see it, I just shouldn't have purchased that fur coat without discussing it with you. You feel left out and in a way, 'put-upon'."
4. Listen actively to what the other person is saying: Do not focus on own personal response to be made.
5. Request feedback from the other person to check patient's own perception and interpretation of the other person's communication; for example,
   "You're giving me the impression that you're totally bored with the movie."
6. Encourage verbalization by verbal and nonverbal means to help other person keep talking; for example,
   "Go on."
   "You were saying?"
   Nodding head.
7. Provide feedback by describing some aspect of the other person's communication and its impact on the patient.
8. Confront other person by describing discrepancies between what he says and what he does.

Evaluation/Outcome Criteria

Patient demonstrates successful communication when he
1. Focuses on appropriate input.
2. Transmits concise, clear, and understandable messages.
3. Utilizes congruent verbal and nonverbal communication.
4. Gives and accepts feedback.
5. Experiences satisfaction with communication.

COPING, INEFFECTIVE INDIVIDUAL*

Definition

The patient is unable to formulate a useful appraisal of the stress, does not have an adequate response repertoire, and does not deploy his coping resources.

Etiology

1. Crisis, situational or maturational
2. Poor self-concept

---

* Material in this section was adapted from McFarland G, Wasli E: Coping-stress-tolerance pattern.[6]

3. Nervous system impairment (*i.e.,* sensory, perceptual, cognitive impairments)
4. Severe pain
5. Conflict
6. Lack of social support system
7. Continued stress over period of time
8. Memory loss or memories of past stressful experiences, particularly negative ones

Defining Characteristics

1. Verbalization of inability to cope or inability to ask for help
2. Inaccurate cognitive appraisal
   a. Inability to recognize source of threat
   b. Inability to redefine or interpret threat correctly
   c. Inability to find meaning for the event
   d. Inability to identify the skills, knowledge, and abilities self has to cope with the threat
   e. Inability to formulate goals or outcomes
   f. Inability to make valid appraisal of the threat in context
3. Inadequate response repertoire
   a. Difficulty in expressing feelings, especially anger, fear, and guilt
   b. Use of behaviors destructive to self or others, such as suicide attempts, aggressive acts towards others, and use of alcohol and illicit drugs
   c. Inability to seek out or to learn new skills and knowledge needed to resolve stress
   d. Inability to deal with tangible consequences of stress
   e. Increasing emotional responsiveness or lack of objective responsiveness
   f. Defensive avoidance of dealing with threatening situations
   g. Lack of assertive behaviors
   h. Impaired communication skills
   i. Lack of palliative skills
4. Inappropriate deployment of coping resources
   a. Inability to develop alternative goals, plans, actions, and rewards
   b. Lack of ability to transfer knowledge and/or skills to actual problem resolutions
   c. Relinquishment of hope and spiritual values
   d. Social withdrawal
   e. Difficulty in using problem-solving skills or decision-making skills
   f. Concerns and/or fears about initiating action
   g. Lack of an appropriate coping response because there is not a cognitive cue to act
   h. Lack of supportive social network
   i. Overuse of certain defense mechanisms, such as denial, projection, distortion, hypochondriasis, fantasy, intellectualization, repression, dissociation, and reaction formation
   j. Use of inappropriate behaviors, such as acting-out, passive aggressiveness, and dependency

5. Inability to recover from stress episode
   a. Overdependence on significant others or professional help or institutions
   b. Nonproductive life-style
   c. Nonperformance of activities of daily living
   d. Lack of functioning in usual social roles
   e. Inertia or apathy
   f. Hypervigilance

Nursing Assessment

1. Identify nature of stress.
2. Identify how patient interprets the stress.
   a. Have patient describe the stress.
   b. Determine emotional intensity and factors involved.
   c. Identify ideas, beliefs, and values that patient uses to interpret stress.
   d. Evaluate knowledge gaps.
3. Assess patient's coping responses:
   a. Actions that deal with objective features.
   b. Actions that involve planning of stress or problem-solving process.
   c. Actions that deal with emotional aspects.
4. Note patient's evaluation of the situation, including the following reactions:
   a. Reactions to knowledge about stress.
   b. Reactions to coping responses.
   c. Reactions to emotional responses.

Goals and Nursing Interventions Including Health Teaching

A. To assist patient in perceiving self as able to cope with stress.

1. Convey trust in patient's ability to act and to struggle.
2. Provide direction and assistance in areas where patient needs help.
3. Assist patient in lowering anxiety level.
4. Identify what patient has done to help self.
5. Promote patient's discoveries of self rather than constantly confronting with reality.
6. Begin with a small piece of reality (*e.g.,* "You can go home with your family this weekend," rather than "Mother does not want you to live at home any more."
7. Avoid interaction that focuses on messages such as, "You *do* have a problem—I *don't.*"
8. Assist patient in understanding the coping process.

B. To develop an objective appraisal of the stress, event, or illness.

1. Explore patient's perception of the event by encouraging description.
2. Provide factual information about the threatening stimulus.
3. Provide preparatory information to any patient who is undergoing new procedures and experiences, especially describing the physical sensations and causes of the sensations.

4. Raise questions, encourage data-gathering, and promote an attitude of openness to new information.
5. Avoid evaluative statements when providing information.
6. Help patient work through unresolved memories of past events using image-based reconstruction.
7. Encourage patient to consult professionals in medicine, social work, and law for assistance in interpretations.
8. Make referral for spiritual counseling to assist client in finding meaning in a situation.
9. Give feedback about reality, especially identifying distortions of reality.

C. To develop an awareness of the emotional reactions to the stress, event, or illness.

1. Give empathetic responses to patient's expressions of feelings to encourage acceptance of these feelings in self.
2. Elicit from the patient what he fears and what makes him angry.
3. Provide factual information about the responses of people to crisis (*e.g.,* anger, depression, withdrawal, the powers of crisis resolution, and the grief-mourning process).
4. Give feedback about observed behavior and the feelings expressed.
5. Assist patient in identifying feelings with names that are acceptable and understandable to him.
6. Assist patient in developing ideas about the relationship of his emotional state and consequent thought patterns and behaviors.
7. Set limits on irrational demands.
8. Assist patient in beginning to deal with emotional reactions by examining relationships.

D. Develop coping responses to the objective features of the stress, event, or illness.

1. Assist patient in identifying and making changes in health behaviors that are necessary because of the stress.
2. Serve as a role model and/or social support when assisting patient in performing activities of daily living.
3. Assist patient in identifying areas in which he can act and exert a reasonable amount of control and areas in which he has little or limited possibility of control.

E. To develop plans and actions in response to the stress, event, or illness.

1. Teach patient skills relevant to problem-solving, decision-making, assertive communication, goal-setting, evaluation, study, palliative coping, relaxation, and help-seeking.
2. Assist patient in identifying coping responses that he is using and other coping responses that are possible.
3. Engage patient in role rehearsal and mental imagery for active social role participation.
4. Encourage socialization and social support.

5. Teach patient to monitor self for noneffective thoughts about self or maladaptive behaviors.
6. Explore past situations in which effective coping behaviors were demonstrated.
7. Teach patient to observe changes in behavior of others as he changes or uses another action.

F. To develop coping responses to the emotional reactions to the stress, event, or illness.

1. Help patient reduce anxiety by using recreational and diversional activities as well as by working through feelings of anxiety.
2. Foster constructive outlets for anger and hostility by teaching warning signs of outbursts, ways to gain self-control, and appropriate ways to express anger.
3. Assist patient in working through denial or other defensive mechanisms or to understand and accept it as a coping response useful at a point in time.
4. Teach patient to observe for coping responses of defensive avoidance and hypervigilance, which may impede decision-making.
5. Encourage an attitude of realistic hope as a way to deal with feelings of helplessness.
6. Teach effect of negative self-reflections and derogatory ideas on emotional reactions.
7. Foster expression of feelings through open communication.
8. Assist patient in mobilizing others for emotional support.
9. Encourage use of more mature mental mechanisms (*e.g.,* humor, sublimation, suppression, and altruism).

G. To evaluate the impact of coping response on the objective aspects, on the emotional distress level, and on plans and actions.

1. Give feedback on patient's behavior in order to make him aware of maladaptive responses that tend to foster dependency, manipulate others, and so on.
2. Confront patient about impaired judgment when appropriate.
3. Assist patient in setting reasonable goals.
4. Provide feedback to patient and assist him in eliciting feedback from others.
5. Assist patient in developing cues for self to indicate whether he is reacting automatically or objectively.
6. Give patient a conceptual model for understanding the event or treatment regimen (*e.g.,* model of emotion, model of stress).

Evaluation/Outcome Criteria
1. Patient can accurately appraise stress.
2. Patient demonstrates adequate emotional and cognitive responses.
3. Patient uses adequate coping resources.
4. Patient resolves stress-producing episode.

COPING, INEFFECTIVE INDIVIDUAL, RELATED TO MATURATIONAL OR SITUATIONAL CRISIS

Definition

1. *Crisis*—A state of disequilibrium resulting from an imbalance between a person's perceived difficulty of a hazardous event and his current coping mechanisms and situational supports to deal with this stressor.
2. *Ineffective individual coping related to maturational crisis*—Maladaptive behaviors and emotional changes occurring as a result of transitional periods during psychosocial developmental periods, which require the person to make many character changes.
3. *Ineffective individual coping related to situational changes*—Maladaptive behaviors and emotional changes occurring as a result of environmental stressors.

General Principles

1. Crisis phases can include
   a. Denial—May last for several hours.
   b. Increased free-flowing anxiety—Activities of normal living continued but with much difficulty. Some hyperactivity or psychomotor retardation.
   c. Disorganization—Activities of normal living limited or ceased. May include severe anxiety, fear, guilt, shame, helplessness, depression, or anger. Preoccupation with current hazardous event and earlier symbolically linked events.
   d. Attempted reorganization—Use of familiar coping mechanisms and situational supports lasting several weeks, if successful. If unsuccessful, may lead to escape mechanisms such as blaming others for difficulty, resulting in unsuccessful crisis resolution.
   e. Local and general reorganization—Lower, same, or improved functioning as compared with precrisis level, usually attained in 6 weeks from onset of crisis.
2. Hazardous events or stressors may represent
   a. Threat to integrity of self or instinctual needs
   b. A real or perceived loss
   c. A challenge
3. Crisis is self-limiting with average duration of 6 weeks. Precipitating event often occurs 10 to 14 days before client comes for assistance.
4. Maladaptive resolution of crisis may lead to lowered level of functioning, suicide, violence, or prolonged mental illness.
5. Crisis offers opportunity for personal growth if successfully resolved.
6. Crisis can occur as individual crisis or family crisis.

Etiology

1. Imbalance between actual/perceived resources and actual/perceived hazardous event
2. Transitional stage of psychosocial development

3. Environmental stressors
4. Inadequate personal resources
   a. Physical disorder
   b. Mental disorder
   c. Memory loss
   d. Sensory impairment
5. Lack of supportive social network
6. Perceptual impairment
7. Impaired thought processes

Defining Characteristics

1. Dysfunctional behavior
2. Inability to perform activities of daily living
3. Disorganization
4. Helplessness
5. Extreme denial
6. Severe anxiety
7. Extreme anxiety (panic)
8. Hyperactivity
9. Psychomotor retardation
10. Depression
11. Guilt/self blame
12. Blaming others
13. Extreme anger
14. Inappropriate deployment of coping resources
15. Physical symptoms

Nursing Assessment

1. What are the current behavioral manifestations? Are any suicidal or homicidal impulses present? What is the current level of role functioning?
2. What is the nature of the crisis? Onset? Intensity and duration of precipitating factor(s) or event(s)?
3. How does patient perceive difficulties?
4. What coping mechanisms and problem-solving skills does patient possess?
5. Are there situational supports available such as family or friends?
6. Does the patient's crisis affect other family members? How?

Goals and Nursing Interventions

A. To reduce level of anxiety to level at which patient can function.

1. Establish rapport through warm, empathic, supportive, caring, trustworthy, nonjudgmental approach.
2. Assist patient in recognizing and expressing feelings such as anxiety, anger, and sadness.
3. Reduce anxiety.
4. Support active grieving process.
5. Offer careful, simple explanations during early crisis phases.

6. Reinforce coping mechanisms used effectively by patient in past to reduce tension.
7. Help patient decrease blaming of others.

B. Achieve realistic perception of precipitating event and subsequent experiences.
1. Ask patient to describe sequence of events in process of adjusting to stressor.
2. Help patient gain understanding of crisis by discussing effect of stressor(s) and link to subsequent behaviors.
3. Offer ego support.
4. Convey to patient that difficulties can be understood, that others have undergone similar problems, and that ways for solving the difficulty can be explored.
5. Focus on present, not past, difficulties.
6. Outline target behaviors and goals for therapy, using feasible patient input.
7. Clearly define problem with patient.
8. Clarify experiences by restating previously unconnected facts.

C. To utilize and increase repertoire of coping skills.
1. Encourage use of existing problem-solving skills.
2. Encourage patient to describe own accomplishments in dealing with crisis.
3. Summarize positive changes during therapy.
4. Promote individual responsibility for problem-solving.
5. Explore and examine alternate ways of coping with stress.
6. Suggest and give direct advice and guidance as needed.
7. Formulate action plan
   a. Use situational supports.
   b. Identify and mobilize use of inner strengths and problem-solving skills.
   c. Develop a number of options for action.

D. To utilize and develop situational supports.
1. Make home visits as needed.
2. Offer information about community resources (*e.g.* residential housing), make referrals, or assist patient in contacting agencies.
3. Provide easy access to therapist, within limits.
4. Encourage and use phone as communication link.
5. Encourage use of and reliance on community supports, social service agencies, or significant others.
6. Reduce patient's dependency on therapist after establishing initial rapport.
7. Share treatment plan with patient.
8. Assist patient in increasing his social sphere.
9. Explore resources known by patient.

Health Education and Prevention

1. Teach patient problem-solving skills
   a. Clearly defining problem.
   b. Generating potential solutions.
   c. Describing projected consequences of proposed solutions.
   d. Selecting best alternative.
   e. Testing behavior or action.
   f. Evaluating results.
   g. Redefining problem, if necessary.
2. Use preventive technique of anticipatory planning, tailored to the patient's unique circumstances; describe potential future crises and possible coping strategies.
3. Provide immediate therapy in crises to reduce disorganization, enhance optimal resolution, and prevent psychopathology.

Evaluation/Outcome Criteria

1. Demonstrates precrisis level functioning.
2. Demonstrates improvement over precrisis level functioning.

COPING, INEFFECTIVE INDIVIDUAL, RELATED TO ORGANIC BRAIN SYNDROME

Definition

Impaired adaptive behaviors, emotional changes, and changes in cognitive functioning due to diffuse or localized cerebral damage.

General Principles

1. Personality traits prevalent before onset of organic brain syndrome often become exaggerated and maladaptive following onset of chronic organic brain disease.
2. Behavioral problems, such as extreme withdrawal, may be evident.

Etiology

Organic brain syndrome

Defining Characteristics

1. Changes in cognitive functioning
2. Loss of memory, especially for recent events
3. Disorientation
4. Confusion
5. Wandering and getting lost
6. Decreased ability to concentrate
7. Inability to meet basic needs
8. Inability to meet role expectations
9. Inability to utilize adaptive behaviors to meet all of life's demands
10. High rate of injury to self if unsupervised

11. Inappropriate use of defense mechanisms
12. Alteration in societal participation
13. Inability to problem-solve
14. Poor social graces
15. Irritability
16. Aggression
17. Projection
18. Ritualism
19. Withdrawal
20. Depressive behavior
21. Poor judgment
22. Altered ability to think, learn, reason, and conceptualize
23. Difficulty in communicating

Nursing Assessment

1. Thoroughly assess mental status of patient
   a. Observe patient's general appearance.
   b. Note any unusual bodily movements.
   c. Observe for unusual speech activity, speech patterns, or use of words.
   d. Assess patient's orientation to time, place, and person.
   e. Assess memory for remote events and especially for recent past events and immediate recall.
   f. Note level and fund of knowledge, ability to calculate, and ability to think abstractly.
   g. Observe presence of altered or abnormal perceptions.
   h. Observe for changes in attitude.
   i. Assess unusual mood or expression of emotions.
   j. Note thought processes and content.
   k. Observe patient's judgment.
   l. Note level of alertness.
2. From patient and significant other(s) find out nature of behavioral changes and when changes were first noted.
3. What supportive interpersonal network is available to the patient?
4. What is patient's personal reaction to his illness?
5. What are significant others' reactions to patient's illness?

Goals and Nursing Interventions

A. To prevent injury.

1. Remove environmental hazards, such as loose rugs and small, movable furniture.
2. Keep furniture in same place.
3. Assist with ambulation as necessary.
4. Observe and assist with nutrition and elimination. May use behavior-modification techniques.
5. Assist with personal hygiene.
6. Use close observation and tact if patient is prone to assaultive behavior. Avoid situations that precipitate assaultiveness.

B. To attain the optimal adaptive functioning of which patient is capable.
1. Communicate to patient that he is still a worthwhile human being.
   a. Be supportive.
   b. Show respect and interest in patient.
   c. Be sincere.
   d. Use active listening.
2. Be aware of special needs and attempt to find ways of meeting them.
3. Provide consistent, nonconfusing, quiet atmosphere.
4. Assist patient in being as comfortable and happy as possible.
5. Involve patient in simple, repetitive activities when he can tolerate this (*e.g.,* simple activities in occupational therapy).
6. Provide a homelike atmosphere within limits of safety.
   a. Allow personal belongings.
   b. Encourage use of own clothing.
   c. Use appropriate music.
   d. Interventions may need to be repeated.
7. Develop a therapeutic milieu that provides for structure and routine.
   a. Provide appropriate level of environmental stimulation, maintaining basic daily routine for patient, as he is able to tolerate.
   b. Carefully assess new experiences introduced into patient's life: Some patients will require more structure in routine.
   c. Provide consistency in attitude and approach.
8. Use touch when appropriate.
9. Reduce competition: Emphasize individual achievement.
10. Increase confidence and self-esteem; encourage patient to utilize strengths and potentials.
11. Encourage activities in which success is reasonable and failure minimal.
12. Involve patient in the planning of his own care as much as possible.
13. Involve friends and relatives in care as much as possible.
14. Provide liberal praise and positive reinforcers for accomplishments. Avoid punishment or negative reinforcers.
15. Approach issue of physical and mental limitations with calm, matter-of-fact acceptance.
16. Use quiet firmness.
17. Do not retaliate in response to poor social graces: Recognize this as symptomatic.
18. Use remotivation group therapy as appropriate.
    a. Goals are
       (1) To remotivate patient and focus on reality.
       (2) To help patient develop pleasant interpersonal relationships.
       (3) To help patient recognize things and people and become more aware and interested in surroundings.
       (4) To assist patient in utilizing strengths and potential of patient.
    b. The steps of remotivation therapy include
       (1) "The climate of acceptance"—patients are introduced and warmly welcomed to group.
       (2) "The bridge to reality"—reading of poetry or article in group.

(3) "Sharing the world we live in"—the topic for discussion is introduced using real objects, pictures, and so on.

(4) "An appreciation of the work of the world"—the patient is encouraged to relate his work and life experiences to topic.

(5) "The climate of appreciation"—pleasure is expressed for the member's attendance.

19. Use reality orientation group therapy as appropriate.

   a. Goals are to reorient person to time, place, person, and things.

   b. Classroom group sessions are first held at third-grade level, in daily, 30-minute periods, for 2 weeks.

   c. Use clocks, calendars, and other educational materials to orient patient.

   d. When progress is evident, raise level of instructional materials to sixth-grade level (optional). Use memory games.

20. Use reminiscing group therapy as appropriate.

   a. Goals are

   (1) To help patient identify and share accomplishments, tribulations, and viewpoints with others.

   (2) To increase opportunities for socialization.

   (3) To stimulate memories.

   (4) To help patient gain respect and support from group members.

   (5) To provide for recreation.

   (6) To facilitate putting life experiences into an acceptable meaningful whole.

   b. Have patient engage in mild physical exercise prior to group discussion.

   c. Use developmental framework to organize reminiscing.

   (1) Select initial content area for reminiscing.

   (2) Use real objects to facilitate reminiscing (*e.g.,* use maps to talk about birthplace).

   (3) Plan outings with group as part of therapy.

Health Education

1. Teach patient to care for his own activities of daily living, keeping within capabilities.

2. Teach family use of behavior-modification techniques where appropriate.

Evaluation/Outcome Criteria

1. Patient remains free from injury.

2. Patient attains optimal adaptive level of functioning within limits of available capability.

DEPRESSIVE BEHAVIOR

Definition

A universal mode of interacting manifested by sadness, poor self-concept, and inability to act for self; ranges from mild grief to a psychosis.

Etiology

1. Genetic factors
2. Hormonal imbalances and/or changes
3. Neurotransmitter dysfunction
4. Social factors
   a. Role loss
   b. Culture change
   c. Alienation from group
   d. Lack of social support
5. Psychological factors
   a. Fears of failing
   b. Empty nest
   c. Guilt
   d. Powerlessness
   e. Anger
   f. Negative thoughts
6. Crisis, situational and maturational (especially involving separation, death, and loss)
7. Cognitive errors; negative ideas of self, world, and the future
8. Disease process
9. Belief that stress, event, or illness is uncontrollable

Defining Characteristics

1. Poor problem-solving skills
2. Limited interactions
3. Poor personal hygiene
4. Lack of energy for normal activity
5. Affect flat, sad
6. Suicidal ideation
7. Loss of interest in sex
8. Lack of meaning in life
9. Decrease in social activities
10. Physical complaints
11. Sleep disturbance
12. Verbalization of feelings of worthlessness, hopelessness, helplessness
13. Frequent crying spells
14. Change in appetite or weight
15. Confusion, disorientation

Nursing Assessment and Ongoing Observations

1. Ascertain whether there has been
   a. A recent loss of significant other
   b. An insult to self-esteem
   c. A change in sexual or socioeconomic status
2. Determine extent of withdrawal from family and friends.
3. Identify person with whom the patient feels he can talk.
4. List physical complaints and identify actions taken by patient to cope with them.

5. Note changes in physical complains and determine relationship to level of anxiety.
6. Determine patient's current sleep pattern and inquire what might help extend the period of sleep, if short.
7. Observe current eating pattern and potential for weight loss.
8. Note verbal indications of appetite.
9. Identify which activities patient does for himself.
10. Note recurring thought content and verbalizations (*e.g.*, thoughts about self-worth, fear, worries; expressions of worthlessness, hopelessness, helplessness).
11. Determine suicide potential. It is increased as patient becomes agitated or experiences loss of significant person.
12. Determine homicidal potential. It is increased as patient becomes agitated.
13. Observe changes in coping strategies or ability to plan activities for the day.

Goals and Nursing Interventions

A. To meet basic needs while reducing pervasive feelings of worthlessness, hopelessness, and helplessness.

1. Respond to expressions of feelings; for example, if patient states, "I'm no good," or "There is nothing to live for," a response would be, "I understand you feel worthless."
2. Begin to question the statement "I am no good" by responding, "In what area?"
3. Spend time with patient, even though he says nothing.
4. Avoid arguments or making moral judgments regarding what patient should or should not do.
5. Prevent isolation from others.
6. Confront irrational demands.
7. Use firmness when patient hesitates to do things for himself.
8. Encourage physical activity.
9. Set realistic limits on behavior.
10. Assist patient in setting small goals and experiencing success.
11. Assist him as needed in areas of self-care deficits, such as personal hygiene.

B. To redefine ideas of self or the situation or to expand coping strategies.

1. Set limits on physical abuse of self or others.
2. Listen to angry expressions and assist in constructive expression of anger.
3. When patient begins ruminating, redirect him to other activities or ask for further information about a part of the story.
4. Help patient focus on activity that he has to do now rather than on a physical complaint.
5. Support and give positive feedback for the small decisions made by the patient.
6. Set realistic limits on behavior.

Health Education and Prevention

Teach patient
1. To recognize tension within self.
2. To be alert to sad feelings that may be disguised as anger, most frequently associated with loss.
3. To identify the thoughts that occur just before feelings of helplessness, hopelessness, and sadness.
4. To choose a behavior that will help the feeling diminish.
5. To take action in the future if the situation should recur; to identify potentially stressful situations.
6. When to seek professional help.
7. The importance of doing activities.
8. To give self positive directions and rewards.
9. The beneficial effects of exercise on self-esteem.
10. To focus on his accomplishments instead of the things not done or attempted.

Evaluation/Outcome Criteria

1. Makes positive statements about self.
2. Has normal mood pattern.
3. Makes plans that reflect desire to live.
4. Performs activities of daily living.
5. Uses problem-solving skills.

FAMILY PROCESS, ALTERATION IN

Definition

A family experiencing disruption in the structure and functioning of its system.

Etiology

1. Situational transition and/or crises
2. Developmental transition and/or crises
3. Learned patterns of behavior
4. Intrapsychic conflicts

Defining Characteristics

1. Marital conflict
2. Distance among family members
3. Child described as sick one
4. Emotional, physical, or social illness in one spouse
5. Anxiety
6. Close togetherness or severe separateness
7. Disturbed communication (*i.e.,* difficulty in expression and listening to feelings, thoughts, or beliefs)
8. Role reversals (*i.e.,* parent acts as child and child acts as one of the parents)

9. Disturbed decision-making process
10. Inappropriate or poorly communicated rules, rituals, and symbols
11. Little socialization of members into the community
12. Inability to meet needs of its members

Nursing Assessment and Ongoing Observations

1. Listen carefully to descriptions by all family members of the situation and/or crises, conflicts, and so on.
2. Obtain a family history that includes birth, death, marriage, work education, major moves, and illness of all members.
3. Observe family system for role reversals, rules, secrets, ways of communicating, and methods of decision making.
4. Note any scapegoating process.

Goals and Nursing Interventions

A. To develop communication among family members.

1. Act as mediator, being careful not to take sides.
2. Serve as role model in seeking clarification, showing respect, listening to expression of feelings, giving suggestions, expressing opinions, setting limits, making clear statements.
3. Discuss the role of anxiety in disrupting communication and in developing triangles.
4. Act as counsultant as members work at discovering how to improve communication.

B. To achieve effective problem-solving and decision-making in family group.

1. Assist in clarifying the issue that needs to be resolved.
2. Assist members in identifying problems appropriate for the family to discuss and resolve as a group versus problems appropriate for the individual to work on.
3. Teach steps in problem-solving and decision-making processes.
4. Teach the recognition of emotional factors in the process of problem-solving, especially the effects of anxiety.

C. To promote nurturance and growth of family members.

1. Assist in clarifying "I" and "we" statements.
2. Support the trials of new behaviors.
3. Listen to expressions of fear of change.
4. Explore with family potential maturational crises.

Health Education and Prevention

Many of the interventions are teaching family members other ways of dealing with problems and crises.

Evaluation/Outcome Criteria

1. Conflict resolved among family members.
2. Anxiety lessened within family members.

3. Communication becomes clear among family members.
4. Basic needs of family met.
5. Contact with community maintained.
6. Problem-solving skills acquired.
7. Role relationships clarified.
8. Growth of individual family members encouraged.

FEAR

Definition

A feeling of dread related to an identifiable source which the person validates.[5]

General Principles

1. Fear is a response to a real or threatened external danger.
2. The degree of fear is proportionate to the degree of the danger.
3. Physiological reactions to fear can be similar to those experienced during anxiety.

Etiology

1. Definable, specific danger
   a. Natural dangers, such as sudden noise, loss of physical support, or height
   b. Threat to life, such as diagnosis of cancer
2. Sensory impairment
3. Powerful unmet needs
4. Lack of social support
5. Learned response
6. Knowledge deficit
7. Language barrier
8. Psychomotor impairment
9. Physical handicap or impairment

Defining Characteristics

1. Differentiated emotional response to definable specific danger
2. Fright
3. Apprehension
4. Increased tension
5. Jitters
6. Terror
7. Increased alertness
8. Fight behavior (*e.g.,* aggression)
9. Flight behavior (*e.g.,* withdrawal)
10. Concentration on danger
11. Increased heart rate
12. Increased respiratory rate
13. Pupil dilation
14. Increased muscle tension
15. Diaphoresis

Nursing Assessment

1. Identify and observe for source of danger.
2. Observe for physiological changes (see preceding defining characteristics).
3. Observe for behavioral and emotional changes (see preceding defining characteristics).
4. Determine how the danger is perceived by the patient.
5. Identify coping strategies previously used and presently available to patient.
6. Assess for presence of any anxiety.

Goals and Nursing Interventions

A. To reduce or eliminate fear.

1. Help patient identify the danger.
2. Encourage expression of perceptions and feelings.
   a. Utilize appropriate timing for intervention.
3. Facilitate patient's identification of his usual response pattern in coping with fears.
4. Facilitate/teach coping strategies to deal with fear.
   a. Identify source of danger.
   b. Avoid exposure to danger or work around danger, or eliminate danger.
   c. Develop alternative goals.
   d. Develop additional resources and coping strategies.
   e. Utilize problem-solving skills.
   f. Examine perception of source of danger.

Health Education and Prevention

1. Teach patient problem-solving skills
2. Encourage patient to gain more information about situations and external dangers that have been feared in the past.
3. Encourage patient to increase repertoire of coping strategies.

Evaluation/Outcome Criteria

Reduction or absence of fear: Absence or reduction of characteristics that indicate presence of fear (see preceding defining characteristics).

GRIEVING, ANTICIPATORY

Definition

Grieving process taking place prior to a significant actual loss and occurring in preparation for the actual significant loss.

General Principles

1. The significant loss can refer to such potential significant losses as loss of limb through planned surgery, loss of a friend who is planning to move abroad, and the potential death of a significant person who is terminally ill.

2. Behaviors and feelings exhibited and experienced during anticipatory grieving are very similar to those that are experienced during normal grieving.
3. There may be differences between anticipatory grieving and the normal grieving process that follows a significant loss in end-point, hope, acceleration, and ambivalence.
4. Anticipating grieving can be influenced by interpersonal, sociocultural, and psychological variables.
5. Anticipatory grieving can help a person adjust to the actual loss and lighten the burden of grieving after the loss.
6. Anticipatory grieving can also result in negative consequences, such as immediate postmortem depression.
7. Depending on the experience of anticipatory grieving and the responses of significant others in the environment, anticipatory grieving can be either functional or dysfunctional.

Etiology

1. Perceived potential loss of significant person
2. Perceived potential loss of body part
3. Perceived potential loss of body function(s)
4. Perceived potential loss of prized material possession
5. Perceived potential loss of pet animal
6. Perceived potential loss of social role
7. Perceived impending death of self
8. Perceived potential loss of physiopsychosocial well-being

Defining Characteristics

1. Normal grieving upon anticipation of loss
2. Denial of potential loss
   a. Disbelief
   b. Avoidance of focus on loss
3. Physiological symptoms
   a. Emptiness in stomach
   b. Choking sensations
   c. Exhaustion
   d. Decreased appetite
4. Preoccupation with self
5. Disinterest in daily living
6. Anger
7. Guilt
8. Weeping
9. Sense of unreality
10. Social withdrawal
11. Ambivalence
12. Altered communication patterns
13. Altered activity levels
14. Hope for preventing loss

Nursing Assessment

1. What is the significance of the impending loss to the person?
2. What characteristics of normal grieving are present?
3. Are characteristics of dysfunctional grieving present?
4. How do significant others respond to the person who is experiencing anticipatory grieving?
5. To what extent can the person carry out self care, social, and occupational responsibilities?

Goals and Nursing Interventions

A. To engage in constructive anticipatory grieving.
1. Assist the person through the denial phase.
2. Assist in working through anger phase.
3. Provide support during bargaining and depression phases.
4. Assist client to accept reality of potential loss. Offer realistic hope.
5. Encourage good health habits.
6. Be accepting, supportive, and reassuring.
7. See also goal for dysfunctional grieving—to engage in normal grieving.

Health Education and Prevention

1. Teach use of problem-solving skills.
2. Support and assist patient in coping with impending loss.
3. Assess for risk factors related to dysfunctional grieving and provide patient with extra assistance as needed during anticipatory grieving process.

Evaluation/Outcome Criteria

1. Engages in constructive anticipatory grief work.
2. Meets self-care requirements.
3. Is able to fulfill social and occupational responsibilities.

GRIEVING, DYSFUNCTIONAL

Definition

1. *Grieving*—A normal process, which can last up to 1 year, by which a person adaptively adjusts to a significant loss, which includes
   a. Emotional emancipation from significant loss of object, person, or other established patterns of life.
   b. Readjustment to environment.
   c. Development of new relationships, emotional investment in new objects, and so on to restructure new life and achieve personal reorganization.
2. *Dysfunctional grieving*—Person becomes stuck in one phase of grieving, demonstrating excessive emotional reactions or excessive length of time in a phase.
   a. Is unable to attain acceptance phase and successful adaptation to loss.
   b. Can include prolonged, excessive denial; prolonged depression.
   c. Can lead to mental illness, especially clinical depression.

General Principles

1. Normal grieving unaccompanied by mental problems does not usually require psychiatric referral but is facilitated by skilled interpersonal intervention to prevent the occurrence of dysfunctional grieving and such phenomena as postbereavement morbidity.
2. Physical symptoms that do not last long and frequently appear immediately after loss can include
   a. Sighing respirations.
   b. Choking sensation.
   c. Empty feeling in stomach, digestive upsets.
   d. Physical distress.
   e. Shortness of breath.
3. The exact nature of the normal grief reaction may vary from person to person. Stages can include
   a. *Denial*—Patient avoids acceptance of loss, thereby developing a buffer against reality.
      Acts as if deceased is still present or loss has not occurred. Searching behavior.
   b. *Anger*—Channeled toward lost object or person, toward self, or displaced toward other object or person.
      May place blame on health professionals or may misinterpret what is said by them.
   c. *Bargaining*—Last attempt to postpone realization of loss, which may include bargaining with a deity.
      Attempts to negotiate for change in reality.
   d. *Realization of loss*—Full awareness of loss, including meaning and value of person or object to self, awareness of lost or changed roles, realization of new responsibilities and roles.
      Preoccupation with loss.
   e. *Acceptance and reintegration*—Problem-solving behavior initiated relative to loss and concomitant problems and change.
      Restructuring and reordering of life.

Etiology

1. Perceived or actual loss of significant person, animal, or prized possession
2. Perceived or actual loss of, or change in, social role(s)
3. Unexpected or sudden death of significant other
4. Multiple losses with unresolved grief
5. Perceived or actual loss of body function, part, or physiopsychosocial well-being
6. Inadequate social supports
7. Stressful and prolonged anticipated loss
8. Secondary gains from grieving
9. Overidentification or unfinished business with deceased
10. Inability to attend to grieving because of other tasks
11. Dysfunctional grieving of parents (if child)

12. Unconscious maneuvers of family members to control fate or alleviate guilt (if child)

Defining Characteristics
1. Excessive time in any stage of normal grieving
2. Excessive or distorted emotional reactions
   a. Prolonged or excessive denial
   b. Social isolation or withdrawal
   c. Behavior suggesting that loss occurred yesterday
   d. Developmental regression
   e. Extremely low self-esteem
   f. Severe feelings of identity loss
   g. Unabated searching behavior for lost person or object
   h. Excessive idealization of dead person
   i. Excessive guilt and self-blame
   j. Extreme/prolonged hostility toward dead person
   k. Suicidal ideation
   l. Severe hopelessness
   m. Prolonged panic attacks
   n. Prolonged depression
3. Psychosomatic conditions
4. Engaging in self-detrimental activities
5. Delayed emotional reaction(s)

Nursing Assessment
1. Are defining characteristics of dysfunctional grieving present?
2. What is the nature of the loss? When did it occur?
3. How did the patient perceive the loss? Special meaning/value? Significance of loss in relation to patient's perceived and real abilities to meet his own needs?
4. What stage of grieving and behavioral manifestations does patient currently present?
5. What is patient's behavior between actual occurrence of loss and present?
6. How has patient coped with loss in the past? What strengths were demonstrated in coping with loss?
7. Is patient at high risk for dysfunctional grieving? Examples of such patients are those with
   a. Poor relationship with person prior to death.
   b. Social isolation or poor social network.
   c. History of multiple past losses and use of maladaptive coping strategies.
   d. Presentation of a brave, stoic front.
8. What is the nature of the social network present?
9. What is the degree of depression? Are there suicidal tendencies?
10. What are significant others' reactions to patient's response to loss?

Goals and Nursing Interventions

A. To engage in normal grieving.

1. Assist patient through denial phase.
    a. Help patient understand that others respond similarly when grieving a loss.
    b. Be genuine, honest, and realistic about loss.
    c. Permit visual and tactile contact with body of dead when possible.
    d. Use caring tone of voice.
2. Assist patient through anger phase.
    a. Demonstrate tolerance, patience, and empathy.
    b. Permit open expression of feelings. Do not become defensive.
    c. Assist patient in understanding reasons for feelings.
    d. If patient has difficulty in expressing anger, place him with patients who can express feelings openly.
    e. Reassure patient that feelings of guilt are part of the normal grieving process. Assist in working through feelings of guilt.
    f. Encourage patient to work out conflicting aspect of relationship with deceased. Work through any ambivalence.
3. Assist patient through bargaining phase.
    a. Permit patient's need to talk and reminisce about loss through active listening.
    b. Permit expression of feelings and thoughts. Gently point out reality.
4. Assist through realization of loss phase.
    a. Be physically present; offer support and enhance self-esteem.
    b. Offer acceptance and unconditional positive regard.
    c. Correct misinformation about cause of loss.
    d. Reinforce past and present strengths in dealing with difficulty.
    e. Through sympathetic understanding show that crying is acceptable.
    f. Encourage support for patient from family members and friends.
    g. Observe for and monitor depression.
    h. Facilitate review of positive and negative aspects of lost person, object, or life pattern.
    i. Clarify and offer missing factual information.
    j. Use touch to offer support.
5. Assist through acceptance phase.
    a. Explore nature of problems encountered that are linked to loss with patient.
    b. Raise questions regarding next steps in coping.
    c. Assist in thinking through adaptive coping strategies.
    d. Assist or coordinate resources to develop new skills, to make readjustments in life-style, and to make new emotional investments.
    e. Support patient when he is trying out new coping strategies.
6. Do not suppress symptoms of grieving with drugs; use supportive therapeutic intervention.
7. Answer questions directly and tactfully.
8. Orient patient to new aspects of environment in a simple, clear way.
9. Foster environment in which loss can be placed in spiritual context by

engaging patient in religious and spiritual rituals and practices as desired.

10. Be cognizant of the possibility of different stages of grieving occurring among family members. Help patient and family members communicate with each other.
11. Offer extensive support and guidance in performing activities of living during bewilderment experienced immediately after loss.
12. Demonstrate caring and concern, especially immediately after the loss.
13. Encourage patient to seek help and not be "too proud."
14. Use role play as a way to help work through feelings.
15. Do not abandon patient while he is experiencing loss.

B. To resolve dysfunctional grieving.
  1. Apply interventions outlined for normal grieving.
  2. Assist patient in getting through phase in which he is stuck.
     a. Assess present stage of grieving and the current objects or facts that patient still links to the loss.
     b. Use graded flooding approach.
        (1) Present patient with increasing significant facts about, or objects linked to, loss.
        (2) Rework feelings generated.
        (3) Use role play to work through feelings and preoccupations.
        (4) Apply principles of behavior modification, such as rewards for more adaptive behavior.

Health Education and Prevention

  1. Provide anticipatory guidance and support anticipatory grieving.
     a. Assist patient in coping with expected and impending loss.
     b. Encourage open discussion of impending loss and expression of feelings.
     c. Teach use of problem-solving skills:
        (1) Define potential life changes and problems predicted from the loss.
        (2) Develop alternative potential strategies to deal with problems.
        (3) Map out possible consequences of each strategy.
        (4) Prioritize strategies in terms of usefulness for potential problem resolution.
  2. Offer extra assistance in process of grieving to those at high risk for dysfunctional grieving, such as
     a. Those who had a traumatic, difficult relationship with person who is now deceased.
     b. Those who present cheerful, brave, and stoic behavior.
     c. Those who are socially isolated or who have a poorly developed social network.
     d. Those who have a history of multiple past losses and have used maladaptive coping strategies.
     e. Those who perceive their social network as nonsupportive.
     f. Those with very traumatic circumstances surrounding death of spouse

—anger- or guilt-provoking death, unexpected or untimely death.
g. Those with concurrent life crises.
3. Provide psychological intervention to person with loss, especially in bereavement, to reduce potential for dysfunctional grieving.

Evaluation/Outcome Criteria
1. Engages in normal grief work.
   a. Works through phases of normal grieving.
   b. Recognizes reality of loss.
2. Demonstrates reasonable amount of time in phases of grieving.
3. Demonstrates nonexcessive and nonprolonged emotional reactions.
4. Restructures and reorders life constructively.

GUILT
Definition
A mode of interacting manifested by extremely poor self-concept and feelings of having done or the possibility of doing something wrong and the fear of punishment.

Etiology
1. Conflict between ego and superego
2. Unacceptable behavior in past
3. Crisis, situational or maturational
4. Current violation of socially acceptable behaviors
5. Belief system, particularly religious ideas
6. Life pattern

Defining Characteristics
1. Seeks punishment for self
2. Rejects self as a person of worth
3. Constant recalling of events in which self was wrong; repetitive stories
4. Expressions of worthlessness, failure, bitterness
5. Anxiety
6. Social isolation
7. Limited ability to experience pleasure
8. Inability to forgive self
9. Distorted religious beliefs
10. Blaming
11. Suicidal ideation
12. Tendency to be critical of others
13. Anger
14. Depression
15. Undoing
16. Sexual conflicts
17. Tearfulness

Nursing Assessment and Ongoing Observations

1. Ascertain the presence of the shame–guilt cycle. Inhibition and inaction→passivity→sense of failure→shame and fear of rejection and disapproval→aggressive fantasies and impulses→guilt and fear of responsibility, punishment for wrong→inhibition, and so on.
2. Recognize use of defenses
   a. Denial frequently used to deal with shame.
   b. Projection or blaming others frequently used to deal with guilt.
   c. Guilt can be used to deal with shame. Guilt can explain degree of suffering being experienced and therefore give meaning to suffering.
3. Determine the appropriateness of the guilty feelings.
4. Note use of drugs and alcohol because person may begin to use guilt and ideas of punishment to prevent future use.
5. Ascertain religious belief system.
6. Identify recent crisis, particularly one involving loss or failure.

Goals and Nursing Interventions

A. To maintain or enhance sensitiveness to deal with perceived failure.

1. Support expression of feelings.
2. Discuss consequences of not dealing with guilt and shame.
3. Assist patient in identifying the painful feelings of guilt and then in describing the situation in which they were experienced.
4. Support the patient as he accepts the forgiveness of others.
5. Share experiences of self or others in dealing with shame and guilt.
6. Give feedback about the appropriateness of feelings.

B. To offer opportunity to explore feelings and consequences of guilt.

1. Avoid reinforcing patient's belief that he is guilty.
2. Do not argue over moral issues.
3. Refrain from giving or agreeing with "shoulds" or "should nots."
4. Raise questions about conclusions at which patient has arrived.
5. Listen to the expressions of anger and hostility.
6. Encourage patient to accept consequences of actions without a complete devaluation of himself.
7. Be sensitive to other's need to tell the patient to forget it or to be quiet.
8. Accept revelations in matter-of-fact manner because guilt involves intimate, private, and sensitive parts of the self.
9. Avoid giving false reassurance because this may make patient feel more guilty.
10. Discuss patient's need to be a perfectionist.
11. Discuss alienating effects of guilt on interpersonal relationships.

Health Education and Prevention

Teach patient
1. How to think through the feelings of guilt and shame and to determine appropriateness.
2. Consequences of constantly seeking perfection or the approval of others.
3. The shame–guilt cycle.

4. Constructive ways to deal with failure, such as identifying what needs to be changed to avoid a repeated failure.
5. Appropriate ways to apologize or seek forgiveness from others.
6. Thought-stopping techniques.
7. Use of a worry journal and/or specific time to worry.
8. Recognize when others are attempting to manipulate self through use of guilt.

Evaluation/Outcome Criteria

1. Makes positive statements about self and shows forgiveness of self.
2. Reflects more positive beliefs, religious views of God, sin, and so on.
3. Expresses guilt appropriately.
4. Demonstrates a range of feelings, including joy.
5. Demonstrates satisfying interpersonal relationships.

HYPERACTIVE BEHAVIOR

Definition

A mode of interacting manifested by intense activity that interferes with all aspects of living.

Etiology

1. Genetic factors
2. Neurotransmitter dysfunctions
3. Nervous system abnormality (*i.e.,* perceptual disorder, attention deficit)
4. Food sensitivities

Defining Characteristics

1. Excessive motor activity
2. Difficulty in completing a task
3. Destructive tendencies
4. Short attention span, distractibility
5. Inability to perform activities of daily living

Nursing Assessment and Ongoing Observation

1. Determine whether pattern of hyperactivity during the day is related to environmental stresses, presence of certain people, possible biorhythm, or ingestion of certain foods.
2. Identify sleep pattern and determine when it could be extended.
3. Note patient's ability to carry out grooming skills.
4. Collect data related to eating pattern to determine potential for weight loss.
5. Determine presence of learning disability.
6. Ascertain responsiveness to nondemanding situations in contrast to conflict-laden situations.
7. Observe for signs of increasing hyperactivity and loss of self-control.
8. Collect data on the response to varying stimuli.
9. Check relatedness of fatigue and attention-seeking behaviors to hyperactivity.

Goals and Nursing Interventions

A. To reduce responsiveness to environment.

1. Set limits with hyperactivity when it interferes with others or the patient himself.
2. Decrease number of stimuli, including number of people, in the environment.
3. Offer warm baths and showers.
4. Monitor and reduce the noise level.

B. To provide safe environment.

1. Allow for movement of large muscles in safe, noncrowded area.
2. Provide a quiet area as needed.
3. Actively participate in games with patient.
4. Structure activities during the day.
5. Provide for physical safety; patient may be accident-prone.

C. To maintain consistency in relationships.

1. Provide activities and warm relationships to assist in the reduction of anxiety.
2. Refrain from commenting about activity intensity, but intervene directly as needed.
3. Have short, frequent contacts; let patient know you are available.

Health Education and Prevention

Teach patient

1. Some structured, active games, such as volley ball, run-sheep-run, swimming.
2. To focus on one thing for a set period of time.
3. To complete one task before beginning another.
4. The effects of hyperactivity on self and others.
5. To reduce number of stressors in the environment as a way to maintain control.
6. To maintain balanced diet and refrain from stimulants or foods that may increase hyperactivity.

Evaluation/Outcome Criteria

1. Decreases motor activity.
2. Completes tasks.
3. Is able to perform activities of daily living.

IMPULSIVENESS

Definition

A mode of interacting manifested by acts performed with little or no regard for the consequences.

Etiology

1. Life pattern
2. Nervous system abnormality

3. Anxiety
4. Crisis
5. Aggressive and sexual drives

Defining Characteristics

1. Unpredictable behavior
2. Frequently threatening or hurtful to others
3. Disregard for social customs
4. Irresponsible acts
5. Easily frustrated
6. Poor problem-solving skills
7. Disturbed interpersonal interrelationships
8. Restlessness

Nursing Assessment and Ongoing Observations

1. Collect data on scope of impulsive behaviors.
2. Identify controls used by patient.
3. Determine what actions of staff assist patient in using his own controls.
4. Observe for precipitating factors.
5. Watch for changes in impulsive acts, especially any tendency toward suicide or homicide.
6. Note any expressions of responsible behavior.
7. Identify requests for assistance in maintaining control.

Goals and Nursing Interventions

A. To increase patient's awareness of his own limits.

1. Discuss areas of life or specific people with whom patient feels threatened or afraid.
2. Assist patient in protecting himself and others, if he loses control.
3. Recognize patient's need for distance and provide it.
4. Avoid behaviors that contribute to feelings of being controlled.
5. Interrupt any impulsive act; patient may feel guilty or ashamed as a result of the act.
6. Give frequent feedback about observed behavior as a way to increase patient's awareness of it.

B. To encourage patient to talk through problems rather than act on feelings.

1. Discuss angry interactions with others.
2. Point out consequences of impulsive acts.
3. Assist in applying problem-solving process to problems such as where to live or where to find a job.
4. Assist in regaining control of activity level.
5. Help patient increase tolerance for feelings.
6. Set limits on impulsive actions.

C. To guide patient in being responsible for his own actions.

1. Identify with patient the circumstances contributing to impulsive acts.
2. Explore alternative behaviors after each impulsive act.

3. Give positive feedback when responsible behaviors are noted, such as patient identifying how he is feeling and what he plans to do about it.
4. Discuss the consequences of impulsiveness on self.
5. Provide direct commands to assist patient in managing impulses until he is able to problem-solve.

Health Education
Teach patient
1. To describe what is happening in interpersonal situations and then to identify problems that need a response.
2. To solve problems by defining, determining solutions, testing, and evaluating.
3. To ask for help in identifying thoughts and feelings before acting on feelings.
4. To decrease anxiety by exercise, shower or bath, or by other means, such as decreasing environmental stimuli.

Evaluation/Outcome Criteria
1. Demonstrates use of problem-solving skills in actions.
2. Is able to identify consequences of actions.
3. Shows improved frustration tolerance.
4. Conforms appropriately to social norms.

KNOWLEDGE DEFICIT (SPECIFY)
Definition
Lack of information, skill, attitude, behavior, or life experience that would assist patient in managing a health problem or a potential health problem.

Etiology
1. Lack of exposure
2. Lack of recall
3. Information misinterpretation
4. Cognitive limitations
5. Lack of interest in learning
6. Unfamiliarity with information resources
7. Poor self-concept
8. Complexity of knowledge/skill/behavior/attitude needed
9. Cultural determinants
10. Stage of growth and development
11. Individual learning styles

Defining Characteristics
1. Verbalization of problem
2. Request for information or lack of request
3. Inaccurate follow-through of instruction
4. Inappropriate or exaggerated health behaviors
5. Statement of misconception

Nursing Assessment and Ongoing Observations

1. Make an inventory of information, skills, attitudes, and health behaviors needed. (Many patient education plans focus on the health regimen, neglecting life-style changes.)
2. Determine ways patient has learned most effectively in the past.
3. Identify patient's stage of physical and emotional growth and development.
4. Determine the existence of any cognitive deficit.
5. Collect data on the patient and family resources for learning.
6. Observe effects of learning experiences.

Goals and Nursing Interventions

A. To increase needed information, skill, and attitude.

1. Provide for patient's participation throughout teaching-learning process.
2. Support motivation to learn by altering the task, changing the reward system, and helping patient change his perceptions or relationships.
3. Give opportunity for self-direction.
4. Make learning as satisfying and enjoyable as possible.
5. Assist patient in finding meaning in the learning experience.
6. Provide for a transfer of learning from simple to more complex daily living experiences he encounters.
7. Carefully prepare instructional behavioral objectives.
8. Choose a teaching model appropriate to the type of learning need.
9. Develop a teaching plan, including evaluation measures.

Health Education and Prevention

Teach the specific health behaviors as determined by careful assessment.

Evaluation/Outcome Criteria

1. Verbalizes specific information.
2. Demonstrates skill needed.
3. Demonstrates and verbalizes satisfaction with knowledge, skill, behavior, and attitude gained.
4. Attains satisfactory health behavior.

MANIC BEHAVIOR

Definition

A mode of interacting manifested by intense activity, superficial relatedness, aggressiveness, and manipulation.

Etiology

1. Genetic factors
2. Hormonal imbalance
3. Neurotransmitter dysfunction
4. Crisis, maturational or situational
5. Alienation

6. Very strong dependency needs
7. Toxic substance

Defining Characteristics

1. Euphoria
2. Hyperactivity
3. Diminished sleep
4. Disruptive behavior
5. Distractibility
6. Grandiosity
7. Speech pressure
8. Sarcasm
9. Infrequent eating
10. Demanding of responses from others
11. Superficial interpersonal relationships
12. Rapid mood swings
13. Manipulation of others through attacks on their self-esteem
14. Tendency to be entertaining, sociable
15. Nonacceptance of responsibility for self
16. Testing of limits
17. Alienation from significant others
18. Aggressive, injurious behavior

Nursing Assessment and Ongoing Observations

1. Review life events and note any recent rejection by a mother figure.
2. Evaluate responsiveness to the environment because the patient may be hypersensitive to it.
3. Be alert to possible presence of such organic conditions as epilepsy, neoplasm, infections, or metabolic disturbance and reaction to such drugs as steroids, isoniazid, levodopa, or bromides.
4. Ascertain patient's ability to tolerate group interactions.
5. Collect data on sleeping, eating, and activity patterns.
6. Note relationship between eating pattern and weight maintenance.
7. Determine range of hyperactive behavior.
8. Observe for signs of increasing agitation: increased loudness of voice, increased motor activity, increased irritability.
9. Observe use of manipulation.
10. Be alert to the possible alienation of staff from patient.

Goals and Nursing Interventions

A. To assist patient in appropriate expression of feelings and thoughts.

1. Listen to expressions of feelings and beliefs, but set limits if the words are for the nurse's benefit and not true expressions of feeling states or beliefs.
2. Assist patient in accepting his dependency needs as part of self.
3. Encourage more responsibility for self. Do not convey the message, "I am taking care of you" or allow the patient to express the reverse, "You know everything. Take care of me."

B. To assist patient in coping with rejection he may be experiencing in the environment.

1. Provide protection from group response to disruptive behavior in group meetings by limiting these experiences or having staff sit with patient to provide support and control.
2. Set limits, particularly if patient is demanding, threatening, or seductive toward another.
3. Support involvement in limited number of activities to prevent rejection because of poor performance.
4. Respond to verbal abuse in matter-of-fact manner.

C. To develop ways to decrease or control hyperactivity.

1. Define limits and controls with patient.
2. Provide rest periods.
3. Formulate schedule of activities for the day.
4. Protect from overstimulation.
5. Attempt to distract patient as one way to deal with escalating situation.
6. Assist patient in substituting an activity for the purposeless hyper-activity.
7. Avoid any implication of personal rejection.

D. To gain satisfaction from a less adventuresome life-style.

1. Assist patient in dealing with fact of his illness.
2. Provide supervision or assistance with basic grooming activities.
3. Patiently support patient's efforts to be a group member and not the center of attention.
4. Encourage patient to verbalize the things he is not going to participate in with a change in mood.

Health Education and Prevention

Teach patient

1. The importance of taking antimanic medication as well as its side effects, including toxic effects; associated precautions; facts about routine blood levels; and long-term maintenance.
2. The importance of learning to live with a state of mind that is less than constant euphoria.
3. Ways to channel hyperactivity so as not to be disruptive.
4. The importance of caring for health needs during periods of manic behavior (*i.e.,* diet, rest, exercise, fluids, medication).
5. That feelings of grandiosity may interfere with safety of self or may cause one to overspend or overcharge money.
6. To be alert for cues for seeking professional help (*i.e.,* inability to sleep, euphoria, buying sprees, overuse of alcohol, making of fantastic unrealistic plans, fighting, promiscuity).

Evaluation/Outcome Criteria

1. Makes realistic statements about self.
2. Demonstrates normal range of mood patterns.

3. Demonstrates improved interpersonal relationships.
4. Performs activities of daily living.

MANIPULATION

Definition

A mode of interacting resulting in the control of people to meet own immediate desires and feelings of satisfaction over the success of achieving control.

Etiology

1. Low self-esteem
2. Need for power and control
3. Reliance on others instead of self to meet needs
4. Alienation
5. Learned behavior style
6. Anxiety
7. Crisis

Defining Characteristics

1. Demanding behavior
2. Impersonal use of others to achieve own ends
3. Frequent use of flattery, of actions drawing attention to oneself, of seductive behavior, of forgetting, and of exploiting weakness of others
4. Involvement in other people's problems instead of one's own
5. Fear of relating to others
6. Deception
7. Role reversal
8. Lack of frustration tolerance

Nursing Assessment and Ongoing Observations

1. Identify the range of manipulative behaviors being used by the patient.
2. Determine what problems the patient is avoiding.
3. Note what or who becomes the major focus of manipulative behaviors.
4. Observe what situational factors tend to increase the manipulation.
5. Watch for an increase in patient's ability to identify his own feelings and wants.

Goals and Nursing Interventions

A. To decrease feelings of insecurity and unworthiness, thereby reducing exploitation of others.

1. Allow testing of interpersonal limits.
2. Assist patient in changing view of himself as a victim by defining his rights.
3. Help patient clarify what he wants to do as opposed to doing something because another demands it.
4. Be nonjudgmental as patient examines his manipulative behaviors.
5. Give feedback regarding any type of manipulation attempted.
6. Discuss alternative ways of dealing with people, particularly those in authority.

7. Seek times to interact with patient when he is not demanding to be noticed.
8. Avoid rejective and retaliatory behaviors and power struggles because those behaviors decrease self-esteem.
9. Help to delay the immediate satisfaction of every wish or need.
10. Frequently ask patient what is happening now, what feeling is being felt.

B. To develop trust and security in interpersonal relationships.

1. Ensure documentation of nursing care plan in order to foster a coordinated and consistent effort among health team members.
2. Be consistent in following the specified limits.
3. Demonstrate a willingness to admit to mistakes.
4. Clarify reasons for limit-setting and consequences of breaking the limit.
5. Continuously direct patient's attention to his behavior.
6. Assist patient in exploring the meaning of his behavior and avoid attempts to focus on the nurse's activities.
7. Carefully explain and enforce ward or community rules.
8. Demonstrate concern and respect for others, a model he can imitate.
9. Look for opportunities to teach about ways to meet true needs appropriately.
10. Avoid reinforcing manipulative behavior by assigning patient a staff member to answer questions and respond to requests.

Health Education and Prevention

Teach patient

1. Responsibilities of a person in a patient role (*i.e.,* make requests clearly and to one member of team; attend therapies).
2. To outline activities of the day and to concentrate on accomplishing these.
3. How to approach others in order to meet needs.
4. To identify when his needs or requests are met and the interactions in which he was given consideration and respect.
5. To identify family rules and how he can participate in their formulation and how he can abide by them.
6. To set limits on his own behavior.
7. To recognize signs of anxiety and how to relieve this feeling.
8. How to identify his positive behaviors and to reward himself.

Evaluation/Outcome Criteria

1. Decreases use of manipulation.
2. Verbalizes positive ideas about self.
3. Shows acceptance of responsibility for self.
4. Develops satisfying interpersonal relationships.

NONCOMPLIANCE

Definition

The patient chooses not to conform to a therapeutic recommendation.

Etiology

1. Poor relationships with caregivers
2. Lack of understanding
3. Hearing or vision defect(s)
4. Lack of funds
5. Transportation problem
6. Side effects of medication
7. No improvement—decompensation—with treatment
8. Belief system, particularly religious
9. Past negative experiences
10. Lack of social value and/or acceptance
11. Troublesome or annoying task
12. Denial

Defining Characteristics

1. Missing clinic appointments; not taking medications; not following prescribed treatment; not carrying out instructions
2. Questioning the need for further treatment
3. Procrastination
4. Increasing signs and symptoms of recurring disorder
5. Development of complications
6. Drug blood levels that are incongruent with statements of compliance by patient

Nursing Assessment and Ongoing Observations

1. Examine attitudes of significant others regarding the severity of patient's illness and the acceptance of it as a lifetime condition.
2. Collect data on the meaning of the patient's medication, on the act of taking the medicine, and on the act of refusing to take the medication. There may be social, cultural, and religious implications.
3. Determine personal discomfort experienced as result of noncompliance.
4. Identify health needs.
5. Observe consequences of noncompliance with health care system.
6. Note secondary gains sought.
7. Check accuracy of patient's knowledge about medications and psychotherapy.
8. Identify irrational fears and fantasies related to treatment process.
9. Note patient's record in keeping appointments.
10. Watch for expressions of patient's willingness and intent to follow treatment plan.
11. Ascertain behaviors that indicate patient is following health care advice.
12. Determine positive reinforcers of compliance for the patient.
13. Assess knowledge about the disorder, treatment and consequences of no treatment.
14. Determine adequacy of resources to obtain and continue treatment.

Goals and Nursing Interventions

A. To clarify health needs and behaviors required to meet these needs.

1. Reinforce constructive patient decisions concerning his health needs.
2. Support use of educational materials and provide them.
3. Assist in simplifying treatment instructions.
4. Formulate with patient a list of things to be done.
5. Develop a method for patient to monitor his own progress and report to caregiver.
6. Be specific when identifying a behavior that needs changing.

B. To assist in re-establishing a productive relationship with caregiver and health agency.

1. Clarify misunderstanding of any aspect of treatment process.
2. Give feedback about behavior change resulting from not following directions.
3. Demonstrate respect for patient's views of his illness.
4. Provide weekly visits or more frequent contacts to give support when patient is discouraged.
5. Provide consistent interaction with patient.
6. Make a written contract with patient, clearly stating expectations.

C. To explore relationship between emotional needs and noncompliance.

1. Identify noncompliant behaviors and possible reasons for them.
2. Assist in exploration of mistrust and of threats to autonomy as possible emotional issues.
3. Promote decision-making and self-expression in as many areas as possible, such as the time to take medicine and ways to remember appointments.

Health Education and Prevention

Teach patient

1. What to expect from a health care system.
2. What is expected of him in the role of a person receiving help.
3. To use drug information materials.
4. To know about his illness, the treatment, and its prognosis.
5. Problem-solving techniques and coping skills.
6. To deal with social attitudes that affect his treatment needs.

Evaluation/Outcome Criteria

1. Demonstrates compliance with treatment.
2. Uses effective problem-solving skills.
3. Shows tolerance of inconveniences and effects of treatment.
4. Verbalizes knowledge of treatment, goals, and plans.

PHYSICAL SYMPTOMS, INAPPROPRIATE USE OF

Definition

The patient uses physical complaints as a way of meeting life's demands.

Etiology

1. Life pattern
2. Poor self-esteem
3. Crises
4. Intrapsychic conflict
5. Inadequate coping skills
6. Anxiety

Defining Characteristics

1. Numerous physical complaints with no organic bases
2. Overconcern with health
3. Nagging and demanding quality of complaints
4. Poor self-esteem
5. Strained interpersonal relationships
6. Numerous contacts with health professionals

Nursing Assessment and Ongong Observations

1. Note carefully the character, duration and frequency of symptoms.
2. Note the interpersonal or symbolic meaning of the symptoms. Is patient asking to be cared for, to be listened to, to be relieved of particular responsibilities, to avoid an aspect of his environment?
3. Collect data on recent stressful life events.
4. Watch for potential health danger in presenting symptoms, because patients with psychiatric diagnoses may be at high risk for medical illness.
5. Determine which activities of daily living or life goals the symptoms are disrupting.
6. Identify patient's method of dealing with dependency needs: a denial of; a defending against, with extreme independency; an acceptance, with a clinging to others.
7. Examine environment to determine situational context symptoms.
8. Note expressions of anxiety.
9. Differentiate between involvement in activities of living versus preoccupation with physical illness.

Goals and Nursing Interventions

A. To develop ability to express emotional needs more directly.

1. Encourage expression of feelings.
2. Ask patient to describe feelings and thoughts when describing a body symptom.
3. Give feedback in terms of feelings when patient is noted to be free of symptoms and looks relaxed.
4. Assist in describing feelings, such as "feeling better, more relaxed," and help identify what is helpful in achieving that state.
5. Refrain from "doing something" in response to increased complaints as patient's anxiety mounts.

B. To prevent further alienation from others by constant complaints.
1. Redirect interest in body functions to an interest in the environment.
2. Listen to complaints to convey concern and to become knowledgeable in scope of complaints before setting limits on further expression.
3. Discuss consequences of constant focus on various aches and pains.
4. Verbalize how burdensome things must be for the patient.
5. Support patient's efforts to do something for someone else.

Health Education and Prevention
Teach patient
1. Relaxation techniques, such as visualizing vacation scenes, focusing on each body part in a progressive manner and relaxing it, exercise.
2. How to become aware of one's own feelings.
3. The basic emotional needs of people and ways they are met.
4. Consequences of overusing physical symptoms as a way of dealing with emotional needs.

Evaluation/Outcome Criteria
1. Verbalizes fewer physical complaints.
2. Demonstrates improved interpersonal relationships.
3. States appropriate health concerns and takes appropriate actions.
4. Verbalizes positive statements about self.

POWERLESSNESS
Definition
"The perception of the individual that one's own action will not significantly affect an outcome. Powerlessness is the perceived lack of control over a current situation or immediate happening."[5]

General Principles
1. Five bases for personal social power are
   a. Power based on punishment.
   b. Power based on reward.
   c. Power based on one's legitimate role in an organization.
   d. Power based on knowledge.
   e. Power based on personal characteristics.
2. Locus of control influences how a person views a given situation:
   a. Those high in external locus of control perceive situations to be controlled by external factors (*e.g.*, fate).
   b. Those high in internal locus of control view themselves to be more in control of what happens in any given situation.

Etiology
1. Non-growth promoting health care environment
   a. Misuse of rewards
   b. Misuse of punishments
   c. Staff monopoly of important resources

   d. Removal of personal possessions
   e. Invasion of privacy
   f. Abuse of authority
   g. Lack of individuation
2. Repeated interpersonal problems or failures
3. Lack of available social resources
4. Threat to physical integrity
5. Hospitalization
6. Life-style of helplessness
7. Difficulty in accomplishing developmental tasks
8. Weak identity
9. Loss of control over mental ability

Defining Characteristics[5]

A. Severe
1. Verbal expressions of having no control or influence over situation
2. Verbal expressions of having no control or influence over outcome
3. Verbal expressions of having no control over self-care
4. Depression over physical deterioration that occurs despite patient compliance with regimen
5. Apathy

B. Moderate
1. Nonparticipation in self-care or decision-making when opportunities are provided
2. Expressions of dissatisfaction and frustration over inability to perform previous tasks and/or activities
3. Failure to monitor progress
4. Expression of doubt regarding role performance
5. Reluctance to express true feelings, fearing alienation from caregivers
6. Inability to seek information regarding self-care
7. Dependence on others that may result in irritability, resentment, anger, and guilt
8. Failure to defend self-care practices when challenged
9. Passivity

C. Low
1. Increasing passivity
2. Expressions of uncertainty about fluctuating energy levels

Nursing Assessment
1. Watch for signs and symptoms of depression.
2. Determine orientation to time, place, and person.
3. Observe for strengths and limitations in role performance.
4. Note patient's perceptions about situations and outcomes.
5. Note increase in complaints, demands, and refusal to go along with treatment programs.
6. Observe indications of increase in patient's passivity.

7. Watch for increasing isolation, resistance, and rejection.
8. Note degree of dependency on others.
9. Note ability to express feelings.
10. Check areas that patient feels cannot be changed.
11. Evaluate resistance to change in order to determine whether patient is afraid of change or trying to maintain some control over his life.
12. Note involvement in decision-making.
13. Assess internal versus external locus of control.

Goals and Nursing Interventions

A. To increase ability to control his activities and outcomes.

1. Individualize ward routine as much as possible (*e.g.,* times for bathing).
2. Refrain from labeling patient.
3. Protect patient's privacy.
4. Convey the expectation that patient will seek help with problems experienced.
5. Be attentive to the communications given by the patient.
6. Provide for basic needs with acceptance of dependence and with encouragement of individual freedom, choice, and an increase in self-care.
7. Encourage patient to help create a pleasant environment.
8. Maintain patient's interest in his treatment program.
9. Show willingness to change rules to increase independence of patient in hospital.
10. Assist in redefining relationships.
11. Help identify areas that patient can control.
12. Increase number of activities in the community.
13. Provide patient time for being alone.
14. Call patient by full name or name chosen by patient.
15. Assist patient in identifying feelings of powerlessness.
16. Help patient differentiate those situations that can be changed from those that cannot.
17. Help patient set realistic goals for self.
18. Encourage identification and use of strengths and potential.
19. Help patient identify his personal values.
20. Structure opportunities in which patient can succeed.
21. Encourage questions about treatment regimen.
22. Reward for active participation in own care.

Health Education and Prevention

Teach patient
1. Problem solving skills.
2. Relevant information about his illness and treatment.
3. Assertive communication skills.

Evaluation/Outcome Criteria

Patient controls or influences outcomes in current situations:
1. Verbalizes feelings of being in control of situations and outcomes.

2. Demonstrates adequate role functioning and coping skills.
3. Exhibits appropriate mood.

RITUALISTIC BEHAVIOR

Definition

A group of behaviors repeatedly performed in an attempt to manage life demands.

Etiology

1. Anxiety
2. Developmental stage fixation
3. Conflict between superego and ego
4. Underappraisal of effectiveness of own coping skills
5. Unacceptable feelings about self

Defining Characteristics

1. Manifestations of anxiety
2. Repetitive act or thought; inability to control act or thought
3. Overabundance of detail with little notation of feeling
4. Inflexibility

Nursing Assessment and Ongoing Observations

1. Identify level of anxiety.
2. Evaluate for manipulation and suicidal behavior and any relationship between the two.
3. Note situations that tend to increase anxiety and lead to ritualistic acts.
4. Identify changes in the patient's view of himself and in his view of the repetitive thought or act as being alien to him.
5. Collect data on relief from urgency of repetitive act or thought provided by various activities.
6. Identify specific interpersonal relationships and health routines being adversely affected by repetitive thoughts or acts.
7. Observe for the expression of feelings.

Goals and Nursing Interventions

A. To reduce anxiety level and conscious uncomfortableness with ritualistic behavior.

1. Reward acceptable behavior.
2. Provide opportunities to express feelings.
3. Allow performance of ritual without making demeaning remarks or attempting to stop behavior.
4. Be consistent and time-conscious when making contacts and appointments or giving specific care.
5. Offer information about rituals and obsessions in everyday life.
6. Assist patient in increasing range of behaviors to decrease anxiety.
7. Support patient in talking about repetitive thoughts or acts.
8. Be aware of—and take action to decrease—anxiety level aroused in staff.

9. Assist patient in identifying his way of dealing with anxiety and resulting obsessive thoughts, such as being overly nice; washing hands; repeating a phrase; distracting self by singing, counting, praying; leaving immediate area; or avoiding a known trigger.
10. Give feedback about expressions of obsession and assist him in saying directly what he means.

B. To engage in range of normal activities during day.
1. Plan for additional time to complete rituals.
2. Assist in making schedule of daily activities.
3. Provide patient support in completing his activities, particularly any new ones.
4. Reassure and assist in enduring small periods of relaxation and pleasure.

Health Education and Prevention
Teach patient
1. Ways of dealing with anxiety, such as identifying the feeling, controlling thoughts, exercise.
2. Ways of dealing with consequences of ritualistic behavior.
3. Simple games and recreational activities.
4. To engage in normal activities and to allow for extra time for rituals.
5. Problem-solving techniques.

Evaluation/Outcome Criteria
1. Demonstrates less ritualistic behavior.
2. Uses effective anxiety-resolving techniques.
3. Makes positive statements about self.

SELF-CARE DEFICIT: FEEDING, BATHING/HYGIENE, DRESSING/GROOMING, TOILETING

Definition
The patient does not use skills to meet needs for nutrition, elimination, and grooming in a socially acceptable manner.

Etiology
1. Pain
2. Neuromuscular impairment
3. Nervous system impairment
4. Musculoskeletal impairment
5. Crisis, maturational or situational
6. Depression
7. Anxiety

Defining Characteristics
1. Irregular bathing, unshaven face, body odor, unkempt hair, dirty fingernails; disheveled

2. Poor dental hygiene, bad breath
3. Unmade bed, spilling of food on clothes and table, playing with food
4. Sleeping in clothes
5. Disregard for smoking rules; need for direction for simplest activity
6. No energy to carry out activities, minimal talking
7. Defecating and/or voiding on self, in chair, on floor, in public places
8. Incontinence
9. Difficulty in following directions or forming habits
10. Anxiety

Nursing Assessment and Ongoing Observation

1. Make inventory of areas in which help is needed.
2. Determine other psychological needs the patient is meeting by not caring for himself.
3. Observe effects of praise, simple rewards, success, recognition, and group pressure on behavior.
4. Collect data on daily activities before illness.
5. Validate patient's inability to perform whole self-care activity or part(s) of the activity.
6. Identity self-help devices and/or techniques used or needed.

Goals and Nursing Interventions

A. To re-establish a pattern of living without total dependence on others.

1. Give feedback about improvement in care of personal appearance or other activities.
2. Use consistent repetition of health routines as a means of establishing them.
3. Avoid showing rejection or belittlement as patient struggles with changing behavior.
4. Provide remotivation groups.
5. Assist patient in verbalizing what he is doing, as he does it.
6. Communicate belief that patient is able to learn.
7. Identify tasks that patient can do successfully.

B. To assist in caring for self.

1. Supervise daily activities, such as bathing, cleaning of teeth, bedmaking.
2. Make various creams and toilet articles easily available.
3. Give praise when activity is completed.
4. Allow adequate time for carrying out activities.
5. Do not make demands on patient that he cannot fulfill.
6. Offer support and give as needed; take care not to make patient totally dependent on you.

Health Education and Prevention

Teach patient

1. Basic grooming skills (*i.e.,* how to care for own clothing, how to make bed).

2. Table manners (*i.e.,* how to hold silverware, how to ask for more).
3. Toileting skills.
4. Bathing skills.
5. How to ask for assistance.

Evaluation/Outcome Criteria

1. Demonstrates ability to feed self, to bathe and groom self, to dress self, or to toilet self.
2. Resolves crisis or anxiety state.
3. Achieves pain reduction.
4. Experiences pleasure in caring for self.

SELF-CONCEPT, DISTURBANCE IN: BODY IMAGE

Definition

A disruption in the way one perceives one's body.

Etiology

1. Cognitive perceptual factors; inability to adjust to changes in body image
2. Cultural
3. Spiritual
4. Biophysical
5. Developmental

Defining Characteristics

1. Actual change in body structure and/or function
2. Refusal to look at and/or touch body part
3. Concealment or overexposure of body part
4. Altered social interactions
5. Loss of ego boundaries
6. Trauma to nonfunctioning part
7. Inability to accept change in body wall or boundary
8. Negative feeling about body
9. Preoccupation with loss
10. Feelings of hopelessness
11. Fear of rejection by others
12. Depersonalization of body part
13. Refusal to verify actual change

Nursing Assessment

1. What is the patient's perception of change in body function or structure?
2. What are patient's strengths and resources?
3. What is response of significant others to patient's change in body part or structure?
4. What are patient's goals?

Goals and Nursing Interventions
A. To develop realistic, constructive body image.
1. Support and reinforce efforts to improve body image (*e.g.*, grooming, coping with body loss).
2. Encourage self-acceptance.
3. Assist patient during grieving process.
4. Observe for depression and suicide potential.
5. Encourage patient to examine body wall or boundary area.
6. Encourage patient to participate in social activities without hiding or exposing affected body part.
7. Encourage participation in rehabilitative services, per physician order.
8. Facilitate use of support and cosmetic services.
9. Assist patient in regaining control of ego boundary if necessary.

Health Education and Prevention
1. Teach patient to give self positive reinforcements for efforts to reassume daily responsibilities.
2. Inform patient about support and rehabilitation services in the community.
3. Provide information about affected body parts.

Evaluation/Outcome Criteria
1. Maintains a positive, accepting, and realistic body image.
2. Engages in activities of daily living.
3. Develops a constructive, positive life-style.

SELF-CONCEPT, DISTURBANCE IN: SELF-ESTEEM
Definition
Disturbance in the estimate one places on oneself, including one's self-worth, self-approval, self-confidence, and self-respect.

Etiology
1. Repeated negative experiences
2. Attacks on self-confidence, self-respect, self-worth, and self-approval
3. Cognitive perceptual difficulties
4. Threat of regression from behavior or skills appropriate to age (in older children)
5. Threat to daily routine (in younger children); for example, peer relationships, teacher relationships

Defining Characteristics
1. Devaluation of self through criticism
2. Harsh self-judgment
3. Low sense of self-worth
4. Fears, especially of failure
5. Worrying
6. Feelings of disappointment and helplessness

7. Feelings of fragility and inadequacy
8. Minimization of own real strengths and abilities
9. Sense of self-defeat
10. Gap between his perception of what he would like to be or should be and the self as actually perceived
11. Failure to live up to self-expectations
12. Self-contempt
13. Inability to accept self
14. Denial of self-pleasure
15. Disregard for own opinion and opinions of others
16. Hesitancy to offer own opinions and viewpoints
17. Unreasonable, inflexible standards for self
18. Preoccupation with real or imagined past failures
19. Ambivalency
20. Procrastination
21. Self-destructive behavior
22. Use of poor self-esteem for secondary gains
23. Failure to achieve goals
24. Failure to receive approval from others
25. Lack of love and respect from others
26. Poor interpersonal relationships
27. Inability to accept positive reinforcement
28. Lack of follow-through
29. Failure to take responsibility for self-care
30. Expectations of the worst outcome in many situations

Nursing Assessment

1. What is patient's present perception of self?
2. What does the patient think he should be like? Or what would he be like?
3. What are patient's goals and how realistic are they?
4. What standards does patient set for self? Are they realistic?
5. Assess patient's real strengths and potentials. In what ways has patient been successful in the past?
6. Describe patient's interpersonal relationships. Is there a social network with meaningful others with whom the patient relates well?
7. Observe for manifestations of depression.
8. Observe for any combination of defining characteristics.

Goals and Nursing Interventions

A. To increase self-esteem.

1. Avoid judgmental attitude.
    Do not reject patient for expressing negative feelings.
2. Make aware times patient discounts own opinions.
3. Show empathy.
4. Demonstrate unconditional positive regard.
5. Be congruent and genuine.

6. Communicate acceptance of patient as a worthwhile human being.
7. Show interest in and concern for patient.
   Spend time with patient in groups and in a one-to-one nurse–patient relationship.
8. Assist patient in developing the attitude of not always having to be perfect to feel adequate and good about himself.
   Point out that he is as worthwhile as anyone else.
9. Focus on patient's strengths and potential.
   a. Encourage patient to identify and list strengths and potentials.
   b. Discourage emphasis on failure.
   c. Offer experiences of success.
   d. Encourage participation in rewarding and satisfying experiences.
   e. Encourage patient in developing new skills and in initiating activities in which he can be reasonably successful.
   f. Find ways to utilize strengths.
   g. Encourage patient to formulate his own opinion of self and not to rely on opinions of others completely.
10. Encourage patient to participate in group therapy in which the emphasis is to provide support.
    Through principle of universality, help patient recognize that he is not alone in eperiencing fears and failures.
11. Work through feelings of disappointment.
    Problem-solve to seek constructive resolution to problems faced.
12. Encourage patient to begin taking responsibility for own opinions.
13. Have patient list negative qualities and develop plans to change them.
14. Give compliments on neat appearance, activities well done, and other strengths.
    a. Offer positive reinforcers for actual achievements.
    b. Avoid false praise.
15. Accept patient as person regardless of his thoughts or his past failures.
16. Discourage use of poor self-esteem for secondary gains.
17. Encourage good grooming habits and personal appearance.
18. Assist patient in developing defenses against attack on self.
19. Expand patient's self-awareness.
20. Encourage patient to explore feelings, thoughts, and behavior and to examine critically his own behavior.
21. Encourage patient to accept responsibility for own behavior and to evaluate its outcome in relation to the options available.
22. Assist patient in developing solutions to problems and in setting realistic goals and plans.
23. Help patient begin to take action to meet goals.

Health Education

A. Teach patient assertive behavior and communication skills.
1. Characteristics:
   a. Sensitivity to others' feelings
   b. Use of "I" messages

    c. Respect for behaviors, opinions, and rights of others

    d. Consistency of posture, facial expression, tone of voice with verbal communication

    e. Communication of expectations to others

    f. Recognition of negotiation as viable tactic

    g. Firm but gentle; unyielding where appropriate

    h. Use of force used only when and where necessary

    i. No need for threats

    j. Basis in own human rights

    k. Emphasis on learning and competence

2. Components:

    a. Set goals and express to others your honest thoughts and feelings.

    b. Act on set goals in clear, consistent way.

    c. Accept personal responsibility for consequences of actions.

    d. Remain sensitive to rights and feelings of others.

B. Teach patient to give self positive reinforcement.

For example, patient can treat self to dinner after completing something successfully.

Evaluation/Outcome Criteria

Demonstrates positive self-esteem:

1. Accepts self as worthwhile human being.
2. Sets and achieves realistic and meaningful goals.
3. Engages in, and recognizes benefit of, treatment modalities.
4. Uses assertive behaviors and communication skills.
5. Feels competent.
6. Values own opinions and contributions.
7. Engages in constructive behavior.
8. Has constructive social network.

SENSORY/PERCEPTUAL ALTERATION: VISUAL, AUDITORY, KINESTHETIC, GUSTATORY, TACTILE, OLFACTORY

Definition

The patient is experiencing an alteration of perceptions with consequences in all areas of behavior.

Etiology

1. Altered environmental stimuli, excessive or insufficient
2. Altered sensory reception, transmission, and/or integration (*i.e.,* pain, sleep deprivation, diseases affecting neurological system, problems in communication such as language differences, normal aging processes)
3. Chemical alterations (*i.e.,* electrolyte imbalances, lack of O_2 in blood and other alterations in blood composition, CNS stimulants, depressants, hallucinogens)
4. Psychological stress
5. Brain dysfunction

Defining Characteristics
1. Disorientation with respect to time, place, or persons
2. Altered abstraction
3. Altered conceptualization
4. Change in problem-solving abilities
5. Reported or measured change in sensory acuity
6. Change in behavior pattern
7. Anxiety
8. Apathy
9. Change in usual response to stimuli
10. Indication of body-image alteration
11. Restlessness
12. Irritability
13. Altered communication patterns
14. Unpredictability
15. Mumbling to self
16. Talking about unseen objects
17. Looking about in a frightened, guarded manner
18. Unusual interest in television or radio
19. Complaints of headache
20. Withdrawal

Nursing Assessment and Ongoing Observations
1. Collect data on patient's sleep pattern and prebedtime routines.
2. Determine whether hallucinatory experience involves direction to do some harm to people or things.
3. Observe nonverbal behaviors to detect when patient is hallucinating.
4. Note high risk of suicide.
5. Relate hallucinatory experience to possible increase in anxiety, use of alcohol or psychedelic drugs, organic disease, injury, or high fever.
   a. More animal themes are in the hallucinations of patients experiencing alcoholism.
   b. More human content is in the hallucinations of patients experiencing functional psychosis.
6. Determine whether voices are perceived as helpful, threatening, accusing, or terrorizing.
7. Ascertain which basic needs the hallucinatory experience helps the patient satisfy, such as dependence, acceptance, and self-esteem.

Goals and Nursing Interventions
A. To promote acceptance of patient as a valued human being and to assist his understanding that alterations in perceptions are part of his illness.
1. Assist in describing hallucinatory experience.
2. Provide reassurance of safe, secure environment, especially at night when hallucinatory experiences are more frequent.
3. Leave light on at night if this promotes increased feeling of security.
4. Avoid arguments, proving you are right, or making jokes about voices.

5. Refrain from threats or hostile comments because patient is already extremely fearful.

B. To assist in orientation to present reality.
1. Provide orientation to time, place and person as needed.
2. Give clear, simple directions.
3. Validate reality of experience for the patient, rather than unreal aspects.
4. Assist patient in associating increased anxiety levels with increased alterations in perceptions.
5. Give feedback, especially about reality aspects of conversation.
6. Assist him in identifying concrete objects, smells, sounds, and lights in the immediate environment.

C. To provide external controls if patient feels he cannot stop responding to voices.
1. Provide restraints or quiet area if patient is unable to control response to voices.
2. Ask patient to seek assistance from staff in controlling voices.
3. Stay with patient to assure him of being safe.
4. Explain carefully what is happening and what you are doing.
5. Verbalize any actions; do not rely on nonverbal communication because it may be misinterpreted.
6. Help patient use techniques to lower anxiety level.
7. Provide distractors or increase the stimuli in the environment with music, dance, television, games, walks, and so on.

D. To decrease reliance on voices in order to deal with loneliness, anxiety, and fears.
1. Assist patient in becoming involved in activities on clinical unit or in community.
2. Provide opportunities for him to listen to problems and concerns of others.
3. Help patient find labels for feelings he is experiencing.
4. Support patient when he begins to tell the voices "to go away" or "be quiet" or begins to be consciously involved in other activities as a way of coping with them.
5. Provide opportunity for a consistent, supportive relationship.

Health Education and Prevention
Teach patient
1. That hallucinatory experiences can be a part of mental illness.
2. To approach others and not to withdraw when experiencing hallucinations.
3. Ways of dealing with anxiety, such as relaxation techniques, distraction.
4. To expect hallucinatory experience when in stressful environment or when there is a change in routine activities.
5. To refrain from speaking out loud to voices in presence of others in recovery phase of illness.

Evaluation/Outcome Criteria

1. Demonstrates freedom from unusual perceptions.
2. Uses effective anxiety-resolving techniques.
3. Demonstrates effective coping skills to deal with altered perception state.

SEXUAL DYSFUNCTION

Definition

The patient uses sexual behaviors in a socially unacceptable manner as a way of meeting life's demands.

Etiology

1. Life pattern
2. Hormonal imbalance
3. Increased sexual or aggressive drives
4. Anxiety
5. Inadequate coping skills
6. Impaired self-concept

Defining Characteristics

1. Use of sexually provocative remarks; flirtatiousness; attempts to touch and pinch others; hugging and kissing
2. Masturbation in public places; disrobing; exposure of genitals
3. Recitation of sexual activities or fantasies
4. Magical expectations of others
5. Disturbed interpersonal relationships

Nursing Assessment and Ongoing Observations

1. Ascertain meaning of sexual behavior as release of sexual needs or anxiety, aggressive act, fear of loss of identity, powerlessness, means of obtaining punishment, or need for closeness.
2. Note increase of anxiety during period of sexual acting-out.
3. Identify situations in which sexual acting-out occurs.
4. Check medications patient is taking: Sedatives, narcotics, psychotropics, antidepressants, antihypertensives, antispasmodics, and alcohol affect sexual function.
5. Evaluate knowledge and beliefs regarding sexual function.
6. Check patient's current satisfaction with his sex life.
7. Note patient's view of his sex role.

Goals and Nursing Interventions

A. To regain control over sexual impulses.

1. Identify when level of anxiety increases.
2. Openly discuss sexual behaviors to arrive at understanding of meaning and ways to assist in coping.
3. Provide structured, active games.
4. Give feedback about uncomfortableness created in self or others.
5. Discuss appropriate ways in which sexual needs can be met.

6. Point out what behaviors are sexually provocative and set limits.
7. Reassure patient that sexual behavior is not needed to maintain nurse's interest and concern in him as a person.
8. Suggest various activities to assist in controlling impulse.

B. To maintain identity of self as person, man or woman.

1. Provide opportunities to express feelings of impotence or loss of control.
2. Recognize the fear of homosexuality that may be expressed; support patient in his choice of sex role.
3. Assist patient in identifying his areas of strength.
4. Explore meanings of being a man or woman.
5. Discuss and negotiate ways to provide privacy in long-term hospitalization.

Health Education and Prevention

Teach patient
1. Appropriate ways of dealing with sexual impulses (*e.g.,* intercourse with appropriate person at suitable time in proper place; cold showers; vigorous physical activity; masturbation; sublimation).
2. Major structure and function of the reproductive system.
3. The different meanings associated with the sexual act.
4. The effect of certain tranquilizers on sexual drive.
5. Consequences of sexually provocative behavior.
6. Social skills.

Evaluation/Outcome Criteria

1. Demonstrates appropriate sex role behaviors.
2. Shows no inappropriate seductive behavior.
3. Identifies ways to meet sex needs.
4. Seeks satisfying relationships with others.

SOCIAL ISOLATION

Definition

A mode of interacting that is manifested by an avoidance of interpersonal contact and a retreat into one's personal world.

Etiology

1. Developmental stage fixation
2. Life pattern
3. Illness
4. Alienation
5. Crisis, maturational or situational
6. Severe psychological stress
7. Nervous system alteration

Defining Characteristics

1. Isolation from others; seclusiveness; seeming lack of awareness of environment

2. Disregard for social customs relating to interactions
3. Conversation that consists of short phrases; failure to respond verbally to comments or questions
4. Reduced motor activity; sleeping during the daytime
5. Active avoidance of others
6. Poor eye contact
7. Expression of feelings of aloneness and rejection
8. Interests and actions of earlier developmental stage
9. Flat affect
10. Preoccupied appearance
11. Hostility
12. Delusions
13. Hallucinations
14. Minimal participation in activities of daily living

Nursing Assessment and Ongoing Observations

1. Note ways patient is testing interest of staff in him as a person.
2. Determine how he views himself.
3. Identify persons with whom he has established a relationship.
4. Identify what overprotective attitudes and actions of family or staff are affecting his behavior.
5. Note problems in his thinking and perceiving.
6. Observe interactions with others: how, what, when, where, why.
7. Determine which needs are verbally expressed.
8. Identify situations that tend to increase withdrawal.
9. Observe expressions of feelings of safety and security.
10. Watch for increase in willingness to share own thoughts and feelings.

Goals and Nursing Interventions

A. To increase interaction with others and the environment.

1. Be aware of where patient is in the environment.
2. Give verbal acknowledgment of any absence from meetings.
3. Provide ward activities so there is less time for daydreaming.
4. Encourage patient to change environment by going outside for walks or to movies.
5. Encourage group activity, but if patient has a need to withdraw, support this decision.
6. Have a matter-of-fact approach to unrealistic expressions.
7. Expect testing of reality and negative responses.
8. Verbalize needs met through interpersonal contacts.
9. Give feedback about behavior that is not appropriately related to current happenings in environment.
10. Request and expect verbal communication.
11. Give positive feedback when patient reaches out to others.

B. To develop security in interpersonal contacts.

1. Maintain eye contact.
2. Explain self and reason for interaction.

3. Tolerate silences.
4. Assist with physical needs, if appropriate, as way to establish contact.
5. Convey concern about "his silence" or "not knowing his needs" and willingness to talk with him.
6. Offer own reactions to happenings in the environment.
7. Focus on what is occurring now.
8. Support positive opinions of self.
9. Avoid probing questions because they increase anxiety and withdrawal.
10. Carry on a one-sided conversation, if necessary.
11. Reduce tendency of staff to withdraw from patient.

C. To explore meaning of and to reduce withdrawal.
1. Discuss what is conveyed to others by silence.
2. Use nonverbal techniques to encourage communication.
3. Point out the responsibility of each in a relationship.
4. Provide safe atmosphere to discuss fears of rejection and retaliation.
5. Give patient opportunities to discuss perception of himself.

Health Education and Prevention

Teach patient
1. The difference in being assertive, aggressive, and rejecting in communicating with others (also demonstrate).
2. The consequences of withdrawing from others.
3. To begin association with others by contact through structured activities.
4. Importance of seeking social contact or role models.
5. Problem-solving skills.
6. Communication skills.
7. Basic social skills.
8. Assertiveness skills.

Evaluation/Outcome Criteria

1. Participates in group activities.
2. Establishes a few important relationships.
3. Uses effective mechanisms to deal with anxiety.
4. Makes positive statements about self.

SPIRITUAL DISTRESS

Definition

1. *Spiritual*—Encompasses those all-pervasive needs and forces that, if met, can lead to
   a. The formulation of a positive personal meaning and purpose of existence.
   b. The development of meaning in suffering.
   c. A positive, dynamic relationship to a deity characterized by faith, trust, and love.
   d. Personal integrity and self-worth.
   e. A sense of direction in life characterized by hope.
   f. The development of positive human relationships.

2. *Spiritual distress*—"A disruption in the life principle that pervades a person's entire being and that integrates and transcends one's biologic and psychosocial nature."[5]

General Principles

1. Patients may respond to illness with spiritual distress followed by inadequate resolution or adequate resolution and growth.
2. Spiritual beliefs and fulfillment of spiritual needs can help one overcome physical and mental illness and restore health.

Etiology

1. Separation from own religious community or cultural ties
2. Challenged belief and value system
3. Difficulties or stress in life, such as illness
4. Inability to carry out usual religious rituals and practices
5. Unresolved feelings about death
6. Moral/ethical nature of therapy
7. Lost belief in deity and religion
8. Inescapable predicament that appears to have no solution

Defining Characteristics

1. Expresses disillusionment with meaning of life and death and/or belief system.
   a. Asks, "Why did God permit this to happen?"
   b. Jokes about heaven and hell.
   c. Verbalizes inner conflict about beliefs.
   d. Questions reasons for, or meaning of, existence.
   e. Questions meaning of suffering.
   f. Questions moral and ethical implications of therapeutic regimen.
2. Questions relationship with deity.
   a. Wonders, "Can I blame deity?"
   b. Begins to blame deity for illness or other difficulties experienced.
   c. Expresses anger toward deity.
   d. Desire to depend on and trust deity decreases.
   e. Faith in deity or spiritual beliefs decreases.
3. Searches for idols.
   a. Asks, "Where can I find a new deity?"
   b. Changes usual spiritual practices and rituals.
   c. Searches for alternative beliefs.
   d. Expresses conflict or concern about own beliefs or values.
   e. Seeks spiritual assistance.
4. Indicates lack of will to live.
5. Demonstrates restlessness.
6. Experiences loneliness.
7. Shows mild, moderate, or severe anxiety.
8. Has decreased hope.
9. Seems unhappy.

10. Views people as less helpful, fair, or trustworthy, or expresses less concern for others.
11. Becomes withdrawn or silent.
12. Expresses guilt or shame.
13. Experiences sleep disturbances.
14. Blames self.
15. Has somatic complaints.
16. Denies responsibilities for problems.

Nursing Assessment

1. Obtain data based on following questions:
   a. What do you worship?
   b. How do you perceive your relationship with God now?
   c. How does religion or spiritual beliefs influence your life?
   d. In what ways are religion or spiritual beliefs helpful or not helpful to you in your present illness?
      Determine whether religion is viewed as a supportive or unrealistic resource.
   e. What/who offers you strength and hope right now?
   f. What spiritual practices, symbols, rituals, or literature are important or helpful to you? Has being ill affected any of these?
   g. What effect does your present illness have on your spiritual beliefs and needs? What effect do your spiritual beliefs have on your views about your present illness?
   h. Do you need any spiritual assistance now? Tell me what would be helpful to you? Does your spiritual advisor know you are in the hospital? Would you like to have this person contacted?
2. Observe for evidence of spiritual commitment (*e.g.,* religious articles in room; behaviors such as praying and reading Bible; verbalizations about spiritual topics; visits from spiritual advisor.)

Goals and Nursing Interventions

A. To reach adequate resolution of spiritual distress.

1. Permit patient to keep religious articles or spiritual resources, unless harmful to self or other.
2. Permit patient to continue beneficial spiritual practices and rituals as much as feasible.
3. Listen carefully to patient's communication and develop a sense of timing for prayer, or spiritual rituals.
4. Be honest and offer informed understanding.
5. Encourage talk with other patients who have similar spiritual beliefs.
6. Don't attempt to change patient's spiritual affiliation.
7. Contact spiritual advisor for assistance as needed. Share with spiritual advisor information that is necessary and useful in helping the patient.
8. Communicate willingness to talk about spiritual beliefs. Avoid idle curiosity.
9. Develop or support meaning in life or suffering.
   a. Listen nonjudgmentally and with understanding.

   b. Show tolerance, respect, concern, care, and empathy.

   c. Assist patient in recognizing that spiritual longing or a desire to search for meaning in life or suffering is acceptable.

   d. Convey belief that life is worth living.

   e. Support patient's will to live.

   f. Develop nurse–patient relationship in which patient can be comfortable in exploring meaning in life or suffering.

   g. Encourage patient to develop realistic hope and a constructive philosophy that helps deal with suffering.

   h. Assist patient in facing pain or suffering.

10. Share personal strengths and beliefs as one means of offering support and assistance.
11. Determine and discuss aspects of hospitalization or treatment that may run counter to patient's spiritual beliefs.
12. Reaffirm and mobilize patient's own internal resources and strengths.
13. Provide environment in which patient is free to choose and make his own decision about spiritual beliefs and values.
14. Respond naturally to expressed spiritual needs. Don't avoid conversation about spiritual matters.
15. Assist in exploring spiritual concerns and needs and feasible alternatives.
16. Avoid statements that increase conflict or stress regarding beliefs or values.
17. Maintain conversation about spiritual matters at patient's level.
18. Avoid social stereotyping.
19. Help patient make lists of what is important in his life, prioritize list, and develop personal goals.
20. Suggest asking spiritual being for direction in clarifying doubts.
21. Aid patient in substituting positive thoughts for negative ones.

Health Education

Teach patient to

1. Recognize own personal characteristics of spiritual distress—disillusionment, investigation, idolatry, and resolution.
2. Discuss spiritual concerns with concerned significant other(s) and seek support.
3. Discuss concern with spiritual advisor.
4. Seek psychiatric therapy.
5. Continue to seek and use ways to develop or build on a constructive spiritual belief system by
   a. Participating in discussion groups focusing on spiritual concerns.
   b. Attending and participating in religious or spiritual rituals and practices.
   c. Reading relevant literature.

Evaluation/Outcome Criteria

Spiritual distress resolved:

1. Expresses sense of purpose and meaning in life.

2. Expresses positive relationship with deity.
3. Absence of behavioral/mood changes, such as moderate or severe anxiety, unhappiness, withdrawal, guilt or shame, feeling of worthlessness, depression, somatic complaints, and sleep disturbances.

SUBSTANCE ABUSE (ALCOHOL)

Definition

1. Excessive drinking of alcohol, which occurs
   a. At regular daily intervals,
   b. On regular weekend intervals, or
   c. During *binges* (intoxicated for at least 2 successive days) interspersed with periods of nonexcessive drinking.
2. Difficulty in stopping or reducing amount of alcohol used.
3. Pattern of pathological alcohol use extending for at least 1 month.
4. Impaired social or occupational role functioning.

General Principles

1. Warning signs of impending alcoholism include
   a. Early-morning drinking.
   b. Tendency to hide and sneak drinks.
   c. Binges.
   d. Absence from work, especially after days off.
   e. Arguments about drinking.
   f. Loss of appetite.
2. Chronic patterns of pathological use of alcohol include
   a. Excessive daily drinking,
   b. Excessive weekend drinking, or
   c. Binges of daily excessive drinking extending from weeks to months interspersed with periods of sobriety.
3. Depending on severity of problem drinking, patient can develop
   a. *Blackouts*—Amnesia for experiences occurring during intoxicated states.
   b. *Tolerance*—The need for more alcohol to produce the same desired effect.
   c. *Alcohol withdrawal*—Symptoms following reduction or cessation of drinking that can include "morning shakes," delirium tremens, convulsive seizures, fever, perspiration, hallucinations, and alcoholic psychosis, which are relieved by resumption of alcohol intake.
4. Persons suffering from alcoholism experience a higher suicide and accidental injury rate than the normal population.
5. Alcohol abuse can result in physical problems (*e.g.,* hepatitis, cirrhosis of the liver, gastritis, pancreatitis, anemia, brain damage, peripheral neuropathy).
6. Intoxication is defined as blood alcohol levels of 0.1% or higher.

Etiology

1. Psychological
   a. Need to escape personal problems

    b. Need to escape uncomfortable feelings
    c. Increased stress
    d. Over dependency
    e. Low self-esteem
    f. Inadequate self-identity
2. Sociocultural
    a. Family traits
    b. Peer pressure
    c. Social permissiveness
3. Biological
    a. Genetic factors

Defining Characteristics

1. Impaired social functioning
    a. Arrests for inappropriate behavior
    b. Violence when intoxicated
    c. Divorce
    d. Interpersonal difficulties and anxieties
    e. Traffic accidents while intoxicated
    f. Social isolation
    g. Silliness, loudness, boisterousness
    h. Poor judgment
2. Impaired occupational functioning
    a. Interpersonal difficulties with coworkers
    b. Absenteeism
    c. Poor job performance
    d. Loss of job
    e. Loss of economic security
3. Psychological difficulties
    a. Hostility
    b. Suspiciousness
    c. Withdrawal
    d. Depression
    e. Suicidal attempts or threats
    f. Angry overdependency
    g. Difficulty in expressing feelings
    h. Emotional immaturity
    i. Low frustration tolerance
    j. Low self-esteem
    k. Sex role confusion
    l. Perfectionism
    m. Grandiosity
    n. Ambivalence toward authority figures
4. Pattern of pathological alcohol use
    a. Necessity of alcohol for daily functioning
    b. Periods of temporary abstinence or restricted drinking
    c. Inability to stop drinking
    d. Binges

   e. Blackouts
   f. Continued drinking despite affect on physical condition(s)
   g. Use of nonbeverage alcohol
5. Physical problems (*e.g.,* cirrhosis)

Nursing Assessment

1. Obtain data base by asking the following questions:
   a. At what age did you start drinking alcoholic beverages?
   b. When did you first experience problems with alcohol?
   c. When did you have your last drink? Drinking episode? What kind and how much alcohol did you drink daily during this time?
   d. Describe your drinking pattern during the past year.
   e. Has drinking alcohol created any problems for you? On your job? With your spouse, children, or other relatives? Any arrests? Auto accidents? Financial difficulties? Fights? Accidental falls?
   f. How do you view yourself presently?
2. Assess effect of alcohol on physical health status by asking patient the following:
   a. What is your general physical health like?
   b. Do you have any pain in your stomach? Changes in appetite? Changes in bowel habits? Weight changes? Nausea or vomiting? Throat or mouth irritation? Vomited blood?
   c. Are you having any trouble with your heart? Chest pain? Any swelling? Shortness of breath? Chronic coughs? Coughed up any blood?
   d. Any difficulty maintaining your balance? Vision difficulties? Tremors? Seizures? DTs? Blackouts? Hearing or seeing things? Tingling, pain, or numbness in extremities?
   e. Are you taking any medications now?
   f. Have you been treated before for alcohol problems? Describe.
3. Determine whether patient has been experiencing any stress or having any problems that may lead to drinking.

Goals and Nursing Interventions

A. To recognize and accept drinking problem.
1. Permit patient to describe his perception of the problem.
2. Encourage patient to mention those aspects he dislikes about his drinking behavior.
3. Upon offering such a statement, ask patient to elaborate and describe his feelings about this aspect.
4. Do not induce guilt but attempt to have patient tune in to any feelings of remorse stemming from those aspects he dislikes about his drinking.
5. Point out to patient those negative behavioral consequences caused by his problem drinking.
   a. Do not directly attack alibi system used by patient to explain negative consequences.
   b. Do not make patient feel blameworthy.

    c. Ask patient to state again what he dislikes about his drinking behavior.

    d. Point out differences between what he is saying and reality.

6. Deal with drinking stories calmly and matter-of-factly.
7. Observe for suicidal tendencies if there is evidence of depression.
8. Meet protective and safety needs.
9. Accept matter-of-factly, without retaliation, patient criticism and hostility toward staff and institution.
10. Prevent seizures.
11. Promote adequate nutritional and fluid intake.
12. Decrease anxiety.
13. Promote adequate rest and sleep.

B. To improve self-concept and gain personal hope.

1. Avoid punitive attitude. Be nonjudgmental and understanding.
2. Help patient express feelings of helplessness and inadequacy.
3. Demonstrate concern for and interest in patient.
4. Set realistic goals with patient (*e.g.,* encourage sobriety "one day at a time").
5. Avoid communicating expectations of failing; do communicate verbally and nonverbally that patient *can* overcome difficulties and that there is hope.
6. Give patient tasks that can be performed successfully. Increase responsibilities gradually.
7. Identify, verbalize recognition of, and support use of assets and potential.
8. Help patient establish therapeutic interpersonal relationship.
9. Support participation or leadership in groups and activities.

C. To develop adaptive coping strategies and eliminate need to use alcohol as a means of escape.

1. Reduce social isolation.
    a. Serve as a link between patient and attempts to establish relationships with other people.
    b. Support and strengthen family interest.
    c. Teach socialization skills.
    d. Encourage removal from groups that support excessive drinking and encourage the development of new relationships.
    e. Help patient set up social support system in community.
    f. Facilitate patient interaction with other patients through social activities and conversation.
    g. Assist patient in recognizing how behavior influences that of others.
    h. Support use of assertive communication skills.
2. Involve spouse in aspects of treatment program, along with patient, where possible.
3. Confront when responsibilities are avoided.
4. Suggest referral of spouse or adult relatives to Al-Anon and children to Alateen groups.

5. Assist patient in developing and participating in old or new enjoyable activities and interests.
6. Refer to Alcoholics Anonymous.
7. Suggest referral to treatment components, such as family therapy, couples counseling, occupational therapy, recreational therapy, vocational rehabilitation, religious counseling, group therapy, out-patient follow-up treatment program.
8. Assist in reducing anxiety.
9. Involve patient in patient groups in which gripes can be aired and policies for ward living can be drawn up.
10. Ask patient to develop constructive plans for use of time that he usually spent drinking.
11. Use role play to teach patient how to refuse a drink when offered one in a social setting.
    a. Decide whether or not and how much to drink before entering drinking social environment.
    b. Establish eye contact.
    c. Assertively make statement, such as, "No I do not want a drink."
    d. Request a nonalcoholic beverage, if desired.
12. Confront and deal with manipulative behavior.
13. Use firm kindness to deal with unreasonable demands.
14. Encourage self-care.

Health Education and Prevention

Teach patient
1. Principles for prevention of alcohol abuse:
   a. Help patient become aware and learn to distinguish between acceptable and unacceptable drinking (*e.g.,* teach effects of alcohol intake on driving).
   b. Develop "take it or leave it" attitude and decrease emotionalism associated with drinking alcohol.
   c. De-emphasize drinking for its own sake or as a means to escape problems.
   d. Emphasize other activities and integrate drinking only as a secondary activity.
   e. Offer young people opportunities to drink in controlled settings.
2. Principles of behavioral self-control to reduce alcohol abuse:
   a. Instruct patient to keep record of all drinking—type and amount of drink, location and time of drink, what was happening before taking the drink.
   b. Review records at regular intervals with patient. Show patient how to calculate blood alcohol concentrations for each drinking incident.
   c. Teach patient to examine record for antecedents to his drinking incidents.
      (1) Discuss strategies for any possible alteration of these antecedents.
      (2) Discuss strategies for alternative reactions to antecedents, other than turning to alcohol.

    d. Use role play to aid patient in learning new behavioral responses.

    e. Have patient practice new behaviors and reach eventual independence in self-monitoring.

3. Problem-solving skills:

    a. Recognize existence of a problem.

    b. Define nature of problem clearly.

    c. Develop alternatives for solution along with their anticipated consequences.

    d. Select best alternative, use it, and evaluate its results.

Evaluation/Outcome Criteria

1. Ceases alcohol abuse.

    a. Recognizes and accepts history of drinking problem.

    b. Has identified necessary life-style changes.

2. Demonstrates improved self-esteem.

3. Utilizes constructive and adaptive strategies to cope with stress.

4. Engages in adequate occupational role performance.

5. Engages in adequate social role performance.

SUBSTANCE ABUSE (DRUGS)

Definition

Pathological use of a drug(s) characterized by the following:

1. Frequent need and use of drug for personal functioning

2. Difficulty in reducing or stopping amount of drug used

3. Periodic, unsuccessful efforts to stop use of drug

4. Episodes of complications from drug misuse

5. Frequent use of drug(s) causing impairment in functioning for at least 1 month

General Principles

1. Drugs frequently misused include the following:

    a. Barbiturates and other similarly acting hypnotics or sedatives:

        (1) Barbiturates—Butabarbital sodium, hexobarbital, pentobarbital sodium, phenobarbital, secobarbital sodium

        (2) Hypnotics—Paraldehyde, chloral hydrate, methaqualone, ethchlorvynol, flurazepam, glutethimide, methyprylon

        (3) Minor tranquilizers—Oxazepam, diazepam, chlordiazepoxide

    b. Opioids

        (1) Natural opioids—Heroin, morphine

        (2) Synthetics with morphine-like action—Meperidine, methadone

    c. Amphetamine and other sympathomimetics—Amphetamine, methamphetamine, dextroamphetamine, methylphenidate

    d. Cocaine

    e. Cannabis

        (1) Substances derived from cannabis plant or synthetic substances that are chemically similar

        (2) Marijuana, hashish, delta-9-tetrahydrocannabinol (THC).

    f. Hallucinogens—Dimethyltryptamine (DMT), lysergic acid diethyl-amide (LDS), mescaline, and others

    g. Phencyclidine hydrochloride (PCP) or a similarly acting arylcyclohexy-lamine; ketamine (Ketalar), thiophene analogue of phencyclidine (TCP)

2. Biological, sociological, cultural, and psychological factors interrelate to cause and perpetuate drug misuse

3. Problem drug users often have low tolerance for frustration, tension, or anxiety and turn to drugs to escape.

4. The "reinforcer" received from the "high" that is experienced from the use of many drugs often perpetuates drug misuse.

5. The need to belong to a group, with its own unique life-style, may both contribute to and perpetuate drug misuse.

6. Depending on length and severity of drug misuse, as well as nature of drug, any of the following can develop:

    a. Tolerance—The need for more of the drug to produce the same desired effect.

    b. Physical dependence or addiction—Characterized by withdrawal, a syndrome that follows cessation or reduction in drug use and that can include joint and muscle aches, restlessness, inability to sleep, dilated and sluggish pupils, runny nose, chills, fever, perspiration.

    c. Marked physical or psychological deterioration.

Etiology

1. Biological
2. Sociocultural
    a. Subculture life-style and expectations
    b. Peer pressure
3. Psychological
    a. Low tolerance for tension and anxiety
    b. Need to escape
    c. Reinforced "highs"
    d. Emotional immaturity

Defining Characteristics

1. Impaired social functioning
    a. Interpersonal difficulties with family
    b. Interpersonal difficulties with friends
    c. Arrests for inappropriate behavior
    d. Criminal behavior
    e. Traffic accidents
    f. Lack of ability to communicate well
    g. Personal values that conflict with social standards
2. Impaired occupational functioning
    a. Interpersonal difficulties with coworkers
    b. Absenteeism
    c. Difficulty in job performance
    d. Job loss

3. Physical problems*
   a. Malnutrition
   b. Vasculitis
   c. Toxic reactions
   d. Allergic reactions
   e. Nasal septum erosion
   f. Septicemia
   g. Tetanus
   h. Hepatitis
   i. Infective endocarditis
   j. Embolic phenomena
   k. Organic brain syndrome
4. Maladaptive behavior patterns/feelings
   a. Impulsiveness
   b. Irrational behavior
   c. Manipulative behavior
   d. Grandiosity
   e. Withdrawal
   f. Inappropriate expression of anger
   g. Poor self-concept
   h. Mistrust and suspiciousness
   i. Low stress tolerance
   j. High dependency needs
   k. Mood liability
   l. Violence
   m. Depressive behavior
   n. Suicidal attempts or threats

Nursing Assessment

1. What drug(s) was(were) misused most recently? When? How much?
   a. Describe behavior on admission. Assess for depression and suicidal threats and attempts.
   b. Assess physical condition, including nutritional state and habits. Any evidence of withdrawal?
2. What was the pattern of drug misuse during the last month? Kind(s) of drug(s) used? Amounts? Frequency? Source? Effects on personal functioning?
   a. Current role performance in school or on job?
   b. Interpersonal relationships with family and with friends?
   c. Any financial difficulties?
   d. Legal difficulties? Arrests?
   e. Describe general life-style.
3. In what way does patient perceive drug misuse as problematic?
4. At what age did patient start misusing drugs? What kinds of drugs were used? Frequency? Amounts? Effects on personal functioning?
5. What triggers misuse of drugs?

---

* Problems depend on type of drug and length of its use.

6. Do family members or friends misuse drugs? What are family members' attitudes towards patient's misuse of drugs?
7. Has patient received prior treatment for drug misuse? When? Where? Kind of treatment?
8. Assess strengths useful in developing alternative coping patterns.
9. Observe for signs of continued drug misuse.

Goals and Nursing Interventions

A. To meet physiological and safety needs.

1. Assist with activities of daily living as needed.
2. Observe for signs of withdrawal.
3. Eliminate environmental hazards.
4. Use protective measures during controlled withdrawal.
5. Observe for depressive behavior and suicidal threats and attempts.
6. Set limits on behavior harmful to self or others.
   a. Monitor attempts to secure a continuing supply of drugs.
   b. Offer continuous one-to-one observation when patient is unaware of dangers of his own behavior.
   c. Direct patient in reality-oriented activities when needed.
7. Provide planned and structured environment.
8. Use verbal reassurance to "talk down" patient experiencing "bad trips" from LSD.
9. Place patient experiencing "bad trip" from PCP in a quiet environment, protect from danger, and monitor unobtrusively. Do not attempt to "talk down."
10. Provide opportunity to assist, when possible with self-care.
11. Prevent uncontrolled access to drugs.
    a. On admission, search patient and belongings for drugs.
    b. Monitor visitors, as necessary, to prevent access to drugs.
    c. Observe for attempts to secure additional drugs on unit.

B. To develop alternative coping skills and life-style and to reduce or eliminate drug misuse.

1. Assist in reducing manipulative behavior and impulsiveness.
   a. Increase patient's awareness of behavior.
   b. Explore with patient antecedents of behavior.
   c. Explore alternative ways of relating.
   d. Assist patient in testing alternative ways of relating.
   e. Use precaution with patient's manipulative attempts to obtain supply of drugs.
   f. Set limits on manipulative or impulsive behavior harmful to self or others.
   g. Orient patient to rules and regulations of unit as means to communicate expectations.
2. Assist patient in reducing grandiosity.
   a. Do not respond to grandiosity with verbal attack.
      (1) Point out reality, using appropriate timing.
      (2) Do not argue or laugh at grandiose notions.

    b. Reflect feeling or tone accompanying expressions of grandiosity.

    c. Increase patient's awareness of consequences to himself of his grandiosity.

    d. Work with patient to set realistic goals.

    e. Work with patient to develop schedule and method for achieving goals.

    f. Set limits for behavior harmful to self or others.

3. Assist patient in reducing emotional withdrawal from people and improving interpersonal relationships.

    a. Assist patient in finding satisfaction in relating to others.

    b. Involve patient in one-to-one group conversations.

    c. Intervene with social withdrawal.

    d. Assist patient in development of drug-free social network.

    e. Establish positive nurse–patient relationship.

        (1) Demonstrate acceptance.

        (2) Be consistent. Use rules consistently.

        (3) Show a nonjudgmental attitude toward drug misuse.

        (4) Offer positive reinforcement for appropriate interpersonal behavior.

        (5) Offer support as changes in self-identity occur.

        (6) Provide feedback on the consequences of acting-out behavior.

        (7) Set clear, consistent limits on passive-aggressive behavior.

        (8) Guide superficial talk into personal and meaningful conversation.

        (9) Avoid dependency; foster self-reliance.

4. Help patient develop appropriate ways to express and channel feelings.

    a. Encourage and support physical outlet through activities such as team sports.

    b. Help patient recognize and verbalize feelings such as anger, depression, guilt, suspiciousness.

    c. Help patient recognize antecedents to feelings such as anger, depression, guilt, suspiciousness.

    d. Help patient develop connections between feelings and behavior.

    e. Explore with patient adaptive ways to channel feelings of anger, depression, guilt, suspiciousness.

    f. Suggest biofeedback, relaxation training, group therapy, or meditation.

    g. Avoid critical and punitive approach or retaliation.

    h. Discuss with patient how he may be covering up and avoiding feelings through drug misuse.

5. Explore more adaptive coping strategies for dealing with life stressors other than the misuse of drugs.

    a. Discuss with patient his reasons for misusing drugs.

        (1) Discover rewards gained from drugs.

        (2) Explore more adaptive ways to gain these rewards.

    b. Explore patient's perceptions of present problems caused by misuse of drugs.

    c. Encourage former drug abusers (or drug abusers in treatment) to join therapy groups or group counseling. Orient patient to what is expected from him and how to participate in groups.

    d. Counsel about problems that may be faced in living a drug-free role in the community.

    e. Provide opportunities or make appropriate referrals for patient to develop work habits and job skills.

    f. Provide opportunities or make appropriate referrals to develop interests in new hobbies and activities.

    g. Explore social, psychological, and physical consequences of drug misuse.

    h. Help motivate patient to develop a commitment to a drug-free lifestyle.

    i. Differentiate between expressions of real versus exaggerated physical symptoms.

    j. Rebuild self-esteem and self-concept.

    k. Offer opportunities to assume increased responsibility and earn positive rewards.

    l. Use behavior techniques.

    m. Intervene in family addictive cycle.

      (1) Suggest referral to multiple family therapy, individual family therapy, or marital or couple therapy, as indicated.

      (2) Teach development of mutual attitude concerned with prevention methods rather than one of scapegoating and placing blame.

      (3) Observe family member's, especially mother's, expression of death wish for drug misuser.

      (4) Assist families to deal with anxiety related to separation, to sexual conflicts, and to behavior related to drug misuse, such as acting out.

    n. In methadone maintenance program:

      (1) Develop positive interpersonal relationship with patient. Work through resistance to interpersonal involvement.

      (2) Observe for continued misuse of drugs.

      (3) Assist patient in developing new social networks and new lifestyle.

    o. In therapeutic community, foster peer support and pressure to attain behavior that is free of drug misuse.

Health Education and Prevention

1. Encourage family treatment as a preventive modality, especially for any one of the following:

    a. Families experiencing crises

    b. Immigrant families

    c. Families in which one or more of the siblings misuse drugs

    d. Families in which the parents misuse drugs

2. Increase public awareness in all segments of the community of the harmful consequences of drug misuse; e.g.,

    a. Offer preventive drug programs to 10- to 13-year-old youths, including teaching decision-making and assertive communication skills, to help them deal with peer pressure.

    b. Teach parents signs and symptoms of substance abuse.

Evaluation/Outcome Criteria
1. Ceases drug abuse. Recognizes and accepts drug abuse problem
2. Demonstrates improved self-esteem.
3. Utilizes constructive and adaptive strategies to cope with stress.
4. Engages in adequate occupational role performance.
5. Engages in adequate social role performance.

SUICIDE, POTENTIAL
Definition
The existing possibility that the patient will kill himself voluntarily and intentionally.

General Principles
1. About 80% of the persons who commit suicide give some type of clue indicative of the suicide potential.
2. Clues include the following:
   a. Direct verbal clues such as, "I would like to kill myself."
   b. Indirect verbal clues such as, "You'd be better off without me."
   c. Coded verbalizations such as, "How can I give my body to the medical school?"
   d. Behavioral clues such as suicide attempts or sudden psychological improvement in the depressed person.
   e. Situational clues such as notification that cancer has been diagnosed or significant loss.
3. A specific high-lethality suicide plan (*e.g.*, shooting, poisoning) of recent origin in which the person has the resources available increases the potential of suicide.
4. Suicide may be prevented because persons with the potential for suicide do experience ambivalence sometime prior to actual suicide.
5. More suicides occur during the period of improvement following severe depression than during the period of severe depression itself.
6. A person who experiences delusions or hallucinations may respond to voices that, for example, command that patient to kill himself or herself.
7. Suicide occurs most frequently in those over 45 years of age and among adolescents.

Etiology
1. Depression
2. Changing levels of depression
3. Disturbed thought processes
   a. Delusions
   b. Phobias
   c. Disorientation
   d. Impaired judgement
4. Disturbed perceptions; hallucinations
5. Severe stress
6. Severely impaired self concept

    7. Inadequate coping skills
    8. Inadequate or stressful social network
    9. Physiological disorders
        a. Toxic state
        b. Drug/alcohol withdrawal
        c. Chronic organic brain syndrome
    10. Spiritual stress

Defining Characteristics

    1. Directly verbalizing desire to kill self
    2. Indirectly verbalizing desire to kill self
    3. Verbalizing coded desire to kill self
    4. Having history of previous suicide attempts
    5. Putting unusual things in order before going on a long trip
    6. Making a will under extraordinary circumstances
    7. Buying a casket for self at funeral of significant other
    8. Giving away prized possessions
    9. Psychologically overreacting when stressed
    10. Having action plan for harming self
    11. Experiencing hopelessness
    12. Lacking future plans
    13. Having clouded awareness or understanding
    14. Experiencing difficulty with problem-solving
    15. Withdrawing
    16. Being socially isolated
    17. Feeling agitated
    18. Desperately searching for help, attention, and reassurance
    19. Expressing agitated concern over controlling own fate
    20. Obtaining resources that can be used to kill self

Nursing Assessment

    1. What is the nature of the patient's suicidal behavior leading to admission? Method? Clarity of plan? Place? Proximity of other people? Physical results? Actions to reverse physical results or obtain help?
    2. Does patient verbalize desire to die (*e.g.,* "I'm tired. It's no use. No one would care if I died," or "Death would solve everything.")?
        Ask patient the following questions:
        a. Have you thought of committing suicide?
        b. How would you go about doing it?
        c. Do you have the means?
        d. Have you ever attempted to commit suicide?
        e. Has anyone in your family ever committed suicide?
        f. What is the likelihood that you will?
        g. How do you see your future?
    3. Observe patient's nonverbal behaviors: isolating self, collecting harmful objects, making out wills.
    4. Does patient have a history of suicidal behavior?

5. Observe for signs of depression: lack of interest in activities of daily living, insomnia, lack of appetite, sadness, physical complaints, hopelessness.
6. Does patient exhibit impaired judgment that may result from drug abuse?
7. Has patient experienced delusions or auditory hallucinations?
8. Has patient experienced disorientation, memory impairment, confusion?
9. Has patient made any attempts at suicide in the past? Method used? Place? Proximity of other people? Physical results?
10. Does patient show changes in level of depression?
11. Are any physical illnesses present that may be masked by other behaviors?
12. Assess quality of social network.
13. Utilize established scales for assessing suicide potential (*e.g.,* The Los Angeles Suicide Prevention Center Scale for Assessing Suicidal Potential).
14. In evaluating suicide potential, consider the following variables:
    a. Recent loss of significant person, possession, or role
    b. Degree of social isolation and lack of significant others
    c. Previous suicide attempts or self-destructive behavior
    d. Family history of attempted or actual suicide
    e. History of or current mental illness
       (1) Psychoses with hallucinations and/or delusions
       (2) Depression
    f. Age and sex
    g. Physical pain or illness
    h. Perception of suicide as a release or escape
    i. Verbalizations of wish to die with definite plan specified
    j. Lack of religious beliefs
    k. Financial stress
    l. Domestic difficulties
    m. Occupational status
    n. Alcohol or drug abuse
    o. Highly lethal plan with availability of resources

Nursing Goals and Interventions

A. To maintain safety to self.

1. Provide safe environment, which includes freedom from sharp objects and other harmful items.
   Discuss with team members and decide what personal items to remove from patient and what specific environmental hazards to eliminate.
2. Evaluate with team members the necessity for close observation, area restriction procedures, or one-to-one observations for suicide prevention.
3. Observe patient closely; emphasize protective, not punitive, attitude.
4. Set limits in relation to destructive behavior towards self or others.
5. Permit expression of anger and hostility within these limits.
6. Offer support against self-destructive impulses and suggest alternative behaviors.

7. Prevent isolation. Seek out patient.
8. Do not dare patient to carry out a suicidal threat.
9. Assess impact of patient on staff or other patients.

B. To meet activities of daily living.

1. Assist patient in meeting activities of daily living, permitting as much independence as possible and keeping within the boundaries of patient's capabilities.
2. Allow simple decision-making and progress within limitations of patient.

C. To develop adaptive methods to cope with stress.

1. Ask patient to postpone suicidal attempt.
2. Communicate opportunity to re-evaluate the situation when not overwhelmed by desire to die. Point out that other ways are available to cope with what is happening.
3. Identify what patient believes will be helpful to him.
4. Help patient look at positive aspects of living that can be anticipated in the future.
5. Assist patient in identifying when he is experiencing anxiety.
6. Seek ways to lower anxiety in patient.
7. Avoid interpreting remarks such as "I'll kill myself before I do that" as attention-seeking behaviors.
8. Listen with sensitivity to expressions of unworthiness, without insisting that words are false.
9. Avoid imposing own feelings, values, and moral judgments.
10. Convey message that having bad thoughts and making mistakes does not mean one is a "bad person."
11. Assist patient in developing realistic personal goals.
12. Do not use jubilant, cheerful approach.
13. Help patient identify times when angry, sources of anger, and ways to channel anger.
14. Reflect a caring, concerned attitude.
15. Accept patient as a worthwhile person while conveying that self-destructive behavior is not acceptable.

Health Education and Prevention

1. Teach patient life strategy skills to prevent future suicidal threats, attempts, or actual suicides. Help him do the following:
   a. Establish realistic goals. Master daily activities and rely on self as much as possible.
   b. Minimize distraction from immediate desires and self-indulgence by recognizing each day as an opportunity to increase self-confidence and movement toward realistic goals.
   c. Reduce self-doubts about abilities by focusing on the involvement and satisfaction in the task and by maximizing the use of special skills and abilities.

    d. Set a daily schedule, allowing for flexibility, but making the most out of each part of the day.

    e. Be reasonably selfish so that other people's opinions do not prevent accomplishing new or original activities or meeting personal goals.

    f. Learn to recognize fear and anxiety and their effects. Gather information and engage in focused activity to deal with fear. Evaluate the results of the focused activity. Find the best personal formula to reduce anxiety.

    g. Demonstrate courage, persistence, and self-possession to prevent negative feedback from others.

    h. Use personal goals as an overall frame of focus in order to put complex situations into perspective.

    i. Develop relationships through shared objectives and activities. Resist compromising self-identity or trying to remold others in case of differences.

    j. Focus on positive, not negative, thoughts.

    k. Avoid feeling obligated to reveal self to others continually.

    l. Find solitude to gain strength and focus on personal direction.

    m. Recognize that in future stressful situations, feelings of suicide may occur and that talking to someone is an important aspect of prevention. List hot line phone number and other numbers that may be useful in an emergency.

2. Encourage patient to avoid drinking, becoming exhausted, or taking sedatives.

3. Stress importance of taking medications for depression as ordered, especially after discharge from inpatient setting.

4. Teach patient strategies for maintaining control (*e.g.*, walking or resting in bed) when emotional stress increases and to seek professional help when needed.

Evaluation/Outcome Criteria

1. Suicide potential eliminated.

2. Demonstrates adequate coping skills in dealing with stress.

    a. Demonstrates adequate role functioning.

    b. Exhibits appropriate mood.

    c. Verbalizes hope for own future.

    d. Demonstrates positive self-concept.

    e. Establishes meaningful relationships with others.

    f. Expresses feelings appropriately.

SUSPICIOUSNESS

Definition

A mode of interacting manifested by pervasive mistrust of others.

Etiology

1. Genetic factor
2. Neurotransmitter dysfunction

3. Dysfunctional communication in family
4. Fears of loss of autonomy or loss of self-control
5. Crisis, maturational and situational
6. Anxiety

Defining Characteristics

1. Extreme distrust; belief in conspiracy; feelings of being persecuted and misjudged
2. Frequent isolation from others; conveyance of a superior attitude; concern about status and prestige
3. Inflexible thinking
4. Misinterpretation of acts of others followed by an aggressive response
5. Defense of projection
6. Delusions
7. Alienation
8. Distorted religious beliefs
9. Flat affect
10. Hallucinations
11. Personal language
12. Tense, suspicious manner
13. Inability to problem-solve
14. Inadequate social skills
15. Poor interpersonal relationships

Nursing Assessment and Ongoing Observations

1. Determine extent of contact with significant others.
2. Identify areas in which patient accepts help.
3. Examine patient's fear of losing control.
4. Ascertain areas of daily activities and personal hygiene being avoided.
5. Note behaviors that indicate a seeking of relationships with others or continued isolation from others.
6. Observe for clues that patient is hallucinating (*i.e.,* the way he looks and listens to something besides you).
7. Determine if there is a relationship between aggressiveness and the increased expression of suspicion.
8. Collect data on eating pattern.
9. Collect data on sleeping pattern.
10. Observe patient carefully for taking of medication because he may only pretend to take it.

Goals and Nursing Interventions

A. To develop an increasing sense of reality.

1. Give concrete tasks to increase relatedness to reality.
2. Give clear, concise information when answering questions or offering explanations of what is occurring. Avoid whispering.
3. Question gently the beliefs of the patient.
4. Convey understanding of patient's dilemma without arguing about his ideas.

5. Respond to a delusion by stating the theme or feeling symbolically expressed: "It must be very distressing to believe that." Further state, "I have not experienced him as threatening."
6. Give positive feedback when reality is presented in the conversation.
7. Avoid putting patient on the defensive so that he has to protect himself.
8. Refrain from correcting misinterpretations through reasoning. Instead, as a step in assisting patient to analyze the belief, raise doubt by asking a question.
9. Inform patient of schedule changes as soon as possible.

B. To decrease aggressiveness in social contact, which further threatens self-esteem.

1. Make frequent, short interpersonal contacts by minimal number of staff.
2. Assist in identifying people with whom it is appropriate to share thoughts.
3. Discuss consequences of continued suspicion of others on self.
4. Give assurance that the environment is safe.
5. Listen, demonstrating an accepting attitude.
6. Set limits on aggressive acts toward others.
7. Give feedback when patient is noted to be insulting and threatening towards others.
8. Respect patient's privacy.

Health Education and Prevention

1. Teach patient
2. a. To become consciously aware of feelings of suspiciousness and to make an effort to check them out objectively or to act appropriately despite the fear.
   b. The importance of dealing with feelings and personal space and not the whole environment.
   c. Problem-solving as one way of dealing with misinterpretations of reality.
   d. Steps in the formation of a trusting relationship, such as introducing self, spending time with another, being aware of the other's needs, sharing something in common.
   e. To validate perceptions with others.
2. Demonstrate the consequences of suspiciousness.

Evaluation/Outcome Criteria

1. Establishes basic trust level.
2. Participates in activities of daily living.
3. Makes appropriate appraisals of situations and people.

THOUGHT PROCESSES, ALTERATION IN
Definition
The patient experiences impaired cognitive processes with consequences in all areas of behavior.

Etiology

1. Genetic factor
2. Neurotransmitter dysfunction
3. Developmental stage fixation
4. Anxiety
5. Crisis, maturational or situational
6. Central nervous system dysfunction
7. Chemical alteration (*i.e.,* electrolyte imbalances, lack of O_2, and other alterations in blood composition)
8. Aging process
9. Trauma
10. Sleep deprivation
11. Negative thought patternings

Defining Characteristics

1. Inaccurate interpretation of environment
2. Cognitive dissonance
3. Distractibility
4. Memory deficit or problems
5. Egocentricity
6. Hyper/hypovigilance
7. Inability to follow directions
8. Delusions, flight of ideas, disorganization
9. Word salad, neologisms, echolalia, condensations
10. Perseveration
11. Circumstantiality
12. Difficulty in interacting with others, withdrawal, unpredictability
13. Obsessions
14. Decreased ability to grasp ideas
15. Impaired ability to make decisions
16. Impaired ability to problem-solve
17. Impaired ability to reason
18. Impaired ability to abstract or conceptualize
19. Impaired ability to calculate
20. Disorientation to time, place, person, circumstances, and events
21. Ideas of reference
22. Hallucinations
23. Confabulation
24. Altered sleep patterns
25. Inappropriate affect

Nursing Assessment and Ongoing Observations

1. Carefully validate what is thought to be a delusion. Delusion may be of grandeur or persecution, or somatic delusions.
2. Ascertain whether need for power or self-esteem is being met by a delusion or use of neologism or other type of disturbed thought process.
3. Gather precise descriptive data.

Goals and Nursing Interventions

A. To develop ability to correct delusional system.

1. Give feedback concerning a delusion in terms of feeling tone expressed (*i.e.,* the fear it may generate for the patient).
2. Do not expect rational explanations to change the patient's mind and correct the delusion. They may make the patient cling to his thoughts.
3. Refocus conversation to another topic after you have listened carefully to the delusion.
4. Provide experiences in the here and now that patient can talk to others about and have his experiences validated by others.
5. Have daily schedule that stimulates interest in what is occurring in the real world.
6. Protect patient from receiving too many new and stressful experiences too fast.

B. To communicate thoughts more clearly.

1. Seek clarification from patient when something is not understood.
2. Avoid nodding in agreement when being bombarded with word salad or rapid stream of disconnected phrases.
3. Ask patient to speak slowly.
4. Give frequent feedback as to what you understand patient to be saying.
5. State that you are trying to understand and want to understand what is being said.
6. Create a pleasant, friendly atmosphere for conversation to take place in.
7. Give feedback about "crazy talk" and assist patient in saying directly what he means.

Health Education and Prevention

Teach patient

1. Ways to control thoughts (*i.e.,* to distract self from thinking same thought over and over, to become involved in concrete activities).
2. To recognize when thoughts are becoming disorganized (*i.e.,* people are not answering but staring, finding self jumping from subject to subject).
3. To anticipate increased anxiety in a new situation and to think of a way to decrease the anxiety.
4. To check out ideas and thoughts with others.
5. To practice thought-stopping technique.
6. To engage in thought-switching technique.
7. To dispute irrational thoughts.
8. To use problem-solving process.

Evaluation/Outcome Criteria

1. Ceases to have delusions and obsessions.
2. Demonstrates ability to solve problems.
3. Participates in purposeful activities.
4. Becomes oriented to place, person, and time.
5. Reveals normal range of memory.
6. Demonstrates improvement in ability to relate to others.

REFERENCES

1. McFarland G, Naschinski C: Impaired communication: a descriptive study. Nurs Clin North Am 20, No. 4:775–785, 1985
2. Carpenito L: Nursing diagnoses: Application to Clinical Practice. Philadelphia, JB Lippincott, 1983
3. Kim M, McFarland G, McLane A: Classification of Nursing Diagnoses: Proceedings of Fifth National Conference. St Louis, CV Mosby, 1984
4. Task Force of the National Group for the Classification of Nursing Diagnoses. Subcommittee report on definition of nursing diagnosis. The Fourth National Conference on Classification of Nursing Diagnoses. St Louis, April 9–13, 1980
5. Kim M, McFarland G, McLane A: Pocket Guide to Nursing Diagnoses. St Louis, CV Mosby, 1984
6. McFarland G, Wasli E: Coping-stress-tolerance pattern. In Thompson J, McFarland G, Hirsch J et al: Clinical Nursing. St Louis, CV Mosby, 1986

5
Selected Nursing Interventions

BEHAVIOR THERAPY

Definition

The application of treatment techniques based on the behavioral model and on findings from experimental psychological research.

1. Focuses on current and not on historical determinants of behavior.
2. Relies heavily on psychological research to develop treatment techniques.
3. Objectively and operationally specifies treatment in order that techniques can be replicated.
4. Rejects the medical model and the intrapsychic theories.
5. Stresses overt change in behavior as the main factor in evaluating effectiveness of treatment.
6. Reflects a general scientific approach to treatment rather than a particular set of theoretical propositions.

Three Major Conceptual Approaches to Behavior Therapy

A. Stimulus-response (S-R) mediational view

1. Treatment emphasizes stimulus-response pairing evolving from Pavlov's contiguity learning views (*e.g.,* flooding or systematic desensitization techniques—focus on eliminating underlying anxiety sustaining avoidant behavior).
2. *Classical conditioning*—The process in which new stimuli (which precede a response) control or elicit a respondent behavior or reflex response.
   a. A conditioned stimulus or a neutral stimulus can be associated with the unconditioned stimulus that has been eliciting the reflex response.
   b. When the conditioned and unconditioned stimuli are paired, the conditioned stimulus in time elicits the reflex response.
   c. It is important to assess the patient's psychological responses.

B. Cognitive behavior modification

Treatment techniques are based on the assumptions that people create their own unique environments and that maladaptive behaviors result from faulty cognition, thoughts, and beliefs.

1. Therapy focuses on reducing cognitions resulting in maladaptive behavior and replacing them with thoughts and beliefs that foster adaptive behavior.
2. Therapy also uses behavioral methods to alter cognitive processes as practicing and receiving statements about self that foster adaptive behavior.

C. Applied behavioral analysis

Treatment techniques are based on heritage of operant conditioning and experimental analysis of behavior.

1. Treatment emphasizes changing antecedents and consequences in order to change the identified problem behavior.
2. Techniques utilize principles of reinforcement, extinction, stimulus, control, and so on.
3. *Operant conditioning*—The process in which behavior is emitted or controlled primarily by the consequences that follow the target behavior.
4. *Operants*—Behaviors that can be controlled (made stronger or weaker) by the consequences that follow them.
5. *Reinforcers*—Any event that strengthens or weakens a behavior (*i.e.,* increases or decreases the probability that the behavior will occur again).
   a. *Primary reinforcers*—Natural reinforcers such as food, water, and warmth.
   b. *Secondary reinforcers*—Learned reinforcers such as possessions, compliments, money, and smiles.
   c. *Positive reinforcers*—Events or stimuli following a given behavior that increase the occurrence of that behavior.
   d. *Negative reinforcer*—An aversive event or stimuli following behavior that upon its removal increases the occurrence of that behavior.
   e. *Social reinforcers*—Include reinforcers such as praise, smiling, hugging, and nodding, given with sincerity and enthusiasm.
   f. *Punishment*—The application of an aversive event or stimuli or the removal of a positive event or stimuli after a given behavior that decreases the occurrence of that behavior.
6. Considerations in reinforcement
   a. *Contingency*—The reinforcement must be clearly related to the occurrence of the target behavior. The reinforcement may need to be given immediately after the occurrence of the target behavior.
   b. *Use of primary reinforcers*—These reinforcers, such as food and drink, are best used only for those patients who are not very responsive to other reinforces (*e.g.,* patients who experience mental retardation or psychosis).
   c. *Satiation effects*—Occur when a patient has had enough of a given reinforcer; a different reinforcer must then be used.
   d. *Extinction*—The reduction and eventual cessation of a target behavior upon sudden withdrawal of reinforcement.
   e. *Reinforcement schedules*—Rules set up to specify the frequency and timing by which behavior is reinforced.
      (1) *Continuous reinforcement*—Reinforcing each occurrence of a given behavior.

(2) *Intermittent reinforcement*—Reinforcing some, but not all, occurrences of a given behavior.
   f. *Shaping*—Reinforcing small steps toward a goal response rather than waiting to reinforce the goal response when it occurs.
7. *Observational learning*—The process in which behavior can be newly learned or in which the frequency of a previously learned response can be altered by means of observing a model's behavior.
   a. In order to change behavior, patient need only observe model (*i.e.*, the person need not perform the behavior immediately or receive positive reinforcers).
   b. An effective model gains patient's trust and attention and serves as a realistic reference figure, demonstrating plausible standards of behavior for the patient.

General Principles and Goals

1. The goal of behavior modification is to teach the patient new and more adaptive ways to behave.
2. A treatment plan is developed specifically for each patient based on behavioral assessment and functional analysis.
3. Importance is placed on patient practice, when possible, of the desired behavior in his own community environment.
4. The desired behavioral goals are often jointly defined by the patient and the therapist.
5. The desired behavioral goals, as well as the treatment plan to reach them, are outlined to the patient.

Principles of Behavioral Assessment

1. Data about patient's behavior are collected from diverse settings.
2. Behavioral assessment provides both information relevant to the understanding of the behavioral problem (functional analysis) as well as the formation of a treatment plan.
3. Assessment focuses on current, or "here and now," functioning.
4. Evaluation is ongoing throughout treatment so that treatment effectiveness can be determined.

Settings for Conducting Behavioral Assessments

1. Directly observe and record behavior of patient in situ.
2. Observe patient's behavior while he is role playing or participating in staged interactions.
3. Have patient provide self-report of behavior.
   a. Assist patient in providing retrospective self-report.
   b. Encourage patient to monitor self by documenting ongoing self-observations
   c. Note patient reports of behavioral excesses—behaviors that occur too often, too long, and too intensely or that occur at socially inappropriate times.
   d. Note patient reports of behavioral deficits—behaviors that occur too infrequently, not long enough, and with insufficient frequency or that do not occur at expected appropriate times.

4. Interview patient.
5. Interview significant other.
6. Obtain information from health team members.
7. Use appropriate tools—demographic questionnaires, personality inventories, and projective tests.

Elements of Behavioral Assessment

1. Identify patient's primary problem behavior, also referred to as the *target behavior.*
2. Assess patient's objectives for therapy: What is to be different?
3. Analyze the form or topography of the identified primary problem behavior (target behavior).
   a. How frequently and how long does the behavior occur?
   b. Does the behavior occur more frequently during one part of the entire day?
   c. What is the exact nature of the behavior? Does it vary in intensity, in duration, and so on?
4. Observe physiological responses.
5. Analyze the stimulus situation (*i.e.,* the environment in which the behavior occurs).
   a. What are the antecedents that maintain the identified primary problem behavior?
   b. Can a pattern be identified in the environmental stimuli that takes place prior to the occurrence of the target behavior?
   c. What are the consequences of the target behavior that maintain the behavior?
   d. Can a pattern be identified in the environmental stimuli that takes place following the occurrence of the target behavior?
6. Assess collateral factors.
   a. Behavioral strengths: What strengths or potential does the patient have that could be incorporated into the treatment plan?
   b. What limitations does the patient have that need to be considered in developing the treatment plan?
   c. What environmental strengths and limitations can be identified? For example, what kind of support can the patient potentially receive from significant others to help him change his behavior?
7. Identify potential positive reinforcers for the patient that could be incorporated into the treatment plan.
   a. Find out from the patient what he likes to do. A specific reinforcer does not have the same value for everyone.
   b. Observe for any change in preferences. Reinforcers have different value to the patient as situations in his life change, including changes in his mental health.
   c. Strive to identify possible secondary reinforcers for incorporation into the treatment plan. Primary reinforcers, except for extra food, should not be used.
   d. Identify for possible incorporation into the treatment plan secondary reinforcers that can be utilized upon discharge.

8. Identify potential negative reinforcers in the patient's environment that would impede achievement of the desired behavior. Does the spouse, for example, have a stake in maintaining the target behavior?

Treatment

1. Clearly identify the problem behavior to be changed with the patient.
2. As much as feasible, jointly determine with patient the desired behavioral goal—that is, what behavior is desired instead of the identified problem behavior or target behavior.
3. Clearly identify and describe what is expected in the desired behavior.
   a. When necessary, break desired behavior down into steps and teach patient to master each step in sequence.
      (1) Shaping can be used as positive reinforcement for a response that has not yet reached the level of the desired behavioral response.
      (2) In shaping, closer and closer approximations of the desired behavior are reinforced until the desired behavioral response is reached.
      (3) In shaping, the positive reinforcer must be given immediately after the response sought.
   b. Gradually increase the patient's time spent on the desired behavior.
   c. The desired behavioral goal should first be achieved in a nonstressful environment before it is expected in a stressful environment.
4. Use imitation or modeling to demonstrate to the patient the exact steps involved in performing the behavior.
5. Modify or change any environmental conditions that may prevent the desired behavioral goal (*e.g.,* identify any sources of punishment for the desired behavioral goal and eliminate or reduce them).
6. Select positive reinforcers to be used with patient from assessment data.
   a. Activity reinforcers—Going on trips, ground privileges, going for a walk, staying up late, watching TV, listening to radio, sleeping late.
   b. Social reinforcers—speaking with warm tone, laughing with patient, nodding in agreement, smiling, turning face and body towards patient, touching, sitting next to patient, walking together.
   c. Verbal praise of behavior—"Good for you!" "It pleases me when you . . ."
7. At first, reinforce each desired response immediately after its occurrence; if appropriate, tell patient exactly what response is being rewarded.
8. The desired behavioral response can later be reinforced intermittently.
   a. Fixed interval schedule—The same amount of time elapses before the next reinforcer is given for the desired behavioral response.
   b. Variable interval schedule—The amount of time elapsed varies around a mean before the next reinforcer is given for the desired behavioral response.
   c. Fixed ratio schedule—Reinforcers follow a specified number of occurrences of the desired behavior.
9. Avoid using punishment to change behavior because
   a. It teaches patient to avoid person giving punishment as well as to avoid the punished behavior.
   b. It can teach patient to hate person giving punishment.

   c. It can teach patient to lie, hide, and run away in order to avoid punishment.

GROUP THERAPY

Therapeutic Groups

Overall emphasis or goal is re-education, prevention of health problems, development of potentials, and enhancement of quality of life.

1. Emphasize the repressive inspirational approach, in which negative/maladaptive feelings and behaviors are replaced by more constructive ones.
2. Rely heavily on techniques of support, counseling, and re-education.
3. Are frequently self-help groups (*e.g.*, Al-Anon, Alateen, Alcoholics Anonymous, Recovery, Gamblers Anonymous, Parents Without Partners).

Adjunctive Groups

Goal is to encourage perceptual or sensory stimulation, reality orientation, or resocialization. Examples include the following:

1. *Remotivation groups*—Utilize a five-step technique to aid in resocializing withdrawn or regressed patients.
2. *Reorientation groups*—Foster orientation to self, others, and environment and aim to increase the awareness of very disoriented or regressed patients.
3. *Bibliotherapy*—The patient achieves the goals of perceptual stimulation and interpersonal interaction by reading and discussing books, poems, and newspapers.
4. *Music therapy*—Fosters sensory stimulation and getting in touch with feelings as patient listens to music or plays an instrument.
5. *Social skills groups*—Teach basic social skills. Videotaping may be utilized to increase patient's information about self.

Group Psychotherapy Groups

Overall emphasis, or goal, is problem-solving, insight without personality reconstruction, or personality reconstruction.

A. Personality reconstruction

   Major goals are to modify personality, to modify behavior patterns, and to reduce the use of previously used defense mechanisms where indicated.

1. Characterized by an intensive analytic focus on each patient in the group (*i.e.*, each member is analyzed within the group context).
2. Interpersonal problems occurring among group member are worked through with an emphasis on analyzing the historical roots of these problems. Fosters multiple opportunities for catharsis.
3. Group is long-term and membership to new members is closed.
4. An example is analytical group psychotherapy.

B. Insight without reconstruction

   Goal is to help member gain emotional integration and intellectual insight that increases understanding of the problem and decreases maladaptive behaviors without attempting to achieve major personality reconstruction.

1. Characterized by emphasis on interpersonal problems of members in the "here and now."
2. Goals are achieved through analysis of communications and interpersonal relationships with others.
3. Problems are explored in greater depth than in problem-solving groups.
4. Group helps group member gain greater insight about his effect on others, how others affect him in turn, and about alternative behavioral options.

C. Problem solving

Goal is to help group members resolve circumscribed problems and gain problem-solving skills.

1. Characterized by emphasis on circumscribed problems experienced by a group member (*e.g.,* problems associated with discharge, relating to other patients, and coping with the institutional regimen).
2. Goals are achieved by means of isolating individual patient problems for discussion in the group.
3. Group members contribute ideas for resolving a given problem based on their own education or experience or both. The patient may report the results of the implemented plan of action back to the group.

Types of Groups Based on Theoretical Frameworks

A. Client-centered groups

Based on theories of Carl Rogers.

1. *Goals*—Increased awareness and acceptance of oneself and others, self-actualization, self-responsibility.
2. *Role of therapist*— Is nondirective; shows genuineness, unconditional positive regard, and empathy; focuses on being with the individuals in group and on group process.

B. Transactional analysis groups

Based on theories of Eric Berne.

1. *Goals*—Increased insight; reconstruction of personality structure; assumption of self-responsibility; autonomy in spontaneity and intimacy.
2. *Role of therapist*—Identifies ego states, transactions, and games used by members of group and facilitates more adaptive behaviors; relates openly and honestly in a manner that is free from personal games; serves as teacher and facilitator.

C. Interpersonal groups

Based on the theories of Harry S. Sullivan.

1. *Goals*—Increased insight and personality reconstruction.
2. *Role of therapist*—Serves as participant observer, catalyst, and facilitator; supports enhancement of self-esteem; focuses on link between current problems and prior distorted experiences; encourages consensual validation of behavior in order to correct developmental distortions.

D. Psychoanalytic groups

Based on theories of Sigmund Freud.

1. *Goals*—Reconstruction of personality structure.
2. *Role of therapist*—Serves as neutral sounding board and authority figure; listens actively; focuses on analyzing individual in group dealing with transferences, dream content, resistance, and past traumatic relationships and link to present behavior; focuses on needs of group by identifying group processes operant.

E. Gestalt groups

Based on theories of Frederick Perls.

1. *Goals*—Assuming responsibility for self; increasing awareness of personal feelings and behavior; increasing awareness of the behavior and feelings of others; completing unfinished business (*e.g.,* by experiencing past experiences in the present).
2. *Role of therapist*—Confronts, supports, and takes an active role in directing structured exercises; works with individual group member on the "hot seat" in the "here and now."

F. Existential groups

Based on such theorists as Rollo May.

1. *Goals*—fully experiencing and relating to others; self-actualization.
2. *Role of therapist*—shares self intimately with group as whole; nondirective but guiding when appropriate.

Influencing Factors

Factors in group therapy, therapeutic groups, and/or adjunctive groups that facilitate patient's development of more adaptive behavioral patterns include the following:[1]

1. *Universality*—The patient discovers that he is not alone and that others in the group may experience problems similar to his own.
2. *Instillation of hope*—The patient develops hope for his own improvement as he sees others in the group coping more adaptively.
3. *Corrective reexperiencing of the primary family group*—Group experiences provide the patient with the opportunity to work through conflicts stemming from his primary family group.
4. *Information gained*—The group provides the patient with the opportunity to learn about mental health and mental illness.
5. *Altruism*—The patient benefits from being helpful to other group members (*e.g.,* his self-esteem may be improved).
6. *Group cohesiveness*—Group members are attracted to the group with a sense of "we-ness." Patients in the group develop a sense of belonging, acceptance, individual validation, and ability to express, but tolerate, intermember hostility.
7. *Catharsis*—Patient is able to ventilate his emotions.
8. *Imitative behavior*—The patient observes the behavior of others in the group and experiments with the behavior's usefulness for himself.

9. *Gaining socializing techniques*—The group experience provides the patient with the opportunity to acquire social skills.
10. *Interpersonal learning*—The patient displays his behavior and through feedback and self-observation gains understanding of his impact on others and about the opinions others have of him. The patient gains awareness for his own responsibility in developing his interpersonal world.
11. *Existential factors*—The patient experiences being able to "be" with others and to belong to the group.

Characteristics of Effective Groups

1. Problem-solving is frequently evidenced.
2. Creativity and innovation are supported.
3. Conflict is tolerated, examined, and resolved.
4. High levels of trust, open and two-way communication, support, and inclusion facilitate cohesion.
5. The group atmosphere is relaxed and comfortable.
6. Group members participate in the evaluation of the group's functioning.
7. Decisions are made by consensus.
8. Objectives and tasks are clarified and modified to foster group member commitment.
9. Emphasized are the three group functions—internal maintenance, developmental change, and goal achievement.
10. The leadership role changes among group members over time.

Initiating Group Therapy, Therapeutic Groups, and Adjunctive Groups

1. Decide on type of group to be conducted: delineate the major emphasis and group goals. The specificity of the group goals depends on the type of group.
2. In selecting group members for the type of group, consider
   a. The diagnosis and the degree of mental illness of the patient before placing the patient in group therapy as opposed to group psychotherapy.
   b. Potential therapeutic value to patient (*i.e.,* whether the group helps the patient develop more adaptive behavioral patterns).
   c. Patient motivation and willingness.
   d. Factors such as age, sex, intelligence.
   e. The size of the group—depends to some extent on the type of group and the type of patients. A good range is from 6 to 10 members.
3. Select adequate meeting area. It should be adequate size for group and free from interruptions, have good ventilation, and be attractively furnished.
4. Select time and frequency of meeting.
   a. The actual frequency depends on type of group. A common frequency is once per week.
   b. In selecting the time, work around other patient therapies with less flexibility in scheduling, such as industrial therapy.

c. Changes in meeting place, time, and frequency can adversely affect the group process.

Therapist's Role in Preparing Patient for Group Therapy

1. The therapist's role and interventions will be influenced by the type of group, the type of patients, and the therapist's own theoretical orientation.
2. Preparation of patient for group can vary as follows:
   a. Information about time, place, and frequency
   b. Individual therapy followed by group therapy/psychotherapy
   c. Brief individual orientation
      (1) Time, place, frequency
      (2) Purpose of group
      (3) Brief description of group members
      (4) What is expected of patient in group (*e.g.,* attendance)
      (5) Behavior that will not be tolerated
   d. In an open group (one in which new members can be added at any time), assist the new members in feeling comfortable.
      (1) Introduce the new member to the group and have group members introduce themselves.
      (2) Summarize what the group has been currently discussing.
      (3) Facilitate group support of new member. For example, "Mrs. Jones may need our support in becoming a member of this group. We remember how we felt on our first day."

Phases of Group Development

A. Beginning phase
1. Tasks confronting the group members are
   a. Developing a method for achieving the purpose for which they joined the group.
   b. Managing the social relationships so that each member gains a comfortable role for himself.
2. Patient behavioral characteristics include
   a. Seeking to clarify meaning of group therapy and what group membership entails.
   b. Evaluating and testing other group members and seeking viable personal role.
   c. Seeking acceptance, approval, domination, or respect.
   d. Demonstrating dependency on leader and seeking guidance, approval, and direction.
   e. Using restricted and stereotyped communication.
   f. Searching for member similarities.
   g. Providing description of symptoms, medications, and former treatment.
   h. Showing anxiety among members.

B. Second, or middle, phase

Patient behavioral characteristics include

1. Searching for power, control, and dominance.
2. Engaging in conflicts between members and between members and leader.
3. Searching for appropriate amount of personal power; struggling for control.
4. Expressing criticism and negative comments.
5. Giving advice, judgments, and criticism as means of jockeying for position.
6. Expressing hostility and rebellion towards therapist.
7. Engaging in fantasies of getting rid of leader.

C. Third, or termination, phase

Patient behavioral characteristics include

1. Development of group cohesiveness.
2. Increase in self-disclosure and mutual trust.
3. Increased concern about each other and missing members.
4. Appearance of issues of intimacy and closeness among group members.
5. Increased awareness of interpersonal interactions as they evolve in the group.
6. Final movement of the third phase: teamwork and focus on the purpose and work of the group.
7. Feelings about termination (emerge as group comes to the end).

Interventions

A. Beginning phase

1. Serve as a role model to demonstrate behavior expected in group.
2. Discuss with group members what is expected of them in group. Offer structure and direction.
3. Have members introduce themselves.
4. Foster and facilitate interaction.
   a. Do not permit monopolizing.
   b. Intervene to reduce *social* roles and interaction.
   c. Demonstrate congruence, empathy, and unconditional positive regard.
5. Answer questions in relation to time, place, frequency, and purpose of the group.
6. Do not reinforce group need for dependency on leader.
7. Reduce high anxiety.

B. Second, or middle, phase

1. Permit expression of criticism and hostility toward therapist.
2. Support fragile group member when needed during intermember conflict.

3. Foster and facilitate interaction.
4. Demonstrate congruence, empathy, and unconditional positive regard.
5. Focus on the here-and-now group experiences.
6. Begin to explore themes.

C. Third, or termination, phase
1. Foster and facilitate communication.
2. Encourage exploration of behavior, interactions among members, and topic areas discussed.
3. Provide feedback on group process.
4. Support development of group cohesiveness. Support self-disclosure.
5. Support and encourage problem-solving and working towards group goals.
6. Offer opportunity to work through feelings for loss or addition of group member (especially true for open groups).
7. Encourage members to respond to here-and-now experiences in the group.
8. Work through feelings related to termination of the group.

ADMINISTRATION OF DRUG THERAPY
Areas for Nursing Assessment
The nurse should observe and evaluate
1. Patient perception of the effect that the medication is having on his disorder or health or both.
2. Changes in patient's pattern of eating (*e.g.,* a person begins a 3-day fast and then a fad diet to lose weight) or in the taking of fluids.
3. Changes in elimination pattern, particularly constipation and polyuria.
4. Changes in activity (exercise and work patterns). Resuming daily activities is indication of improvement.
5. Changes in sleep pattern (*e.g.,* patient sleeping most of day).
6. Changes in important interpersonal relationships, including ability to communicate with nurse and others.
7. Changes in ability to function socially (*e.g.,* impotence related to some drug use can be very frightening).
8. Changes in feelings, thought and perception, patterns, and processes (*e.g.,* voices reported returning at night, suspicious manner).
9. Use of other prescribed drugs, alcohol, and street drugs. Many potentially dangerous drug interactions may be averted.
10. Signs/symptoms of other medical problems.
11. Areas for patient education, including readiness for self-medication.
12. Signs/symptoms of side effects, toxicity, tardive dyskinesia. (See specific drug groupings.)
13. Baseline data for future assessment of changes: blood pressure in standing and sitting position, temperature, pulse, respiration, weight, physical examination (done by nurse or physician). The physician generally orders CBC, urinalysis, blood chemistry screens, ECG, and other tests as indicated.

Patient Education

A major responsibility of the nurse is educating patients about their medication. Another group, the National Council on Patient Information and Education (NCPIE), has re-emphasized the importance of patient education and has initiated a "Get the Answers" campaign.

A. People are encouraged to ask full questions concerning their prescriptions:

1. What is the name of the drug and what is it supposed to do?
2. How and when do I take it and for how long?
3. What food or drinks and other medicines or activities should I avoid while taking this drug?
4. Are there any side effects, and what do I do if they occur?
5. Is there any written information available about the drug?

B. Other questions that the patient should ask include the following:

1. How long do I have to wait for the effect?
2. Can I drink alcohol?
3. What is the cost of the medication?
4. What do I do when I forget a dose?
5. Do I need to have my blood pressure or other signs monitored or do I need a blood test?
6. What happens if I just stop taking the medication?
7. How can I tell whether the medication is doing any good?

C. A review of the areas for nursing assessment in administration of drug therapy will assist in identifying other areas of patient teaching.

D. Medication groups

Are effective in teaching psychiatric patients about their medications. The group may have didactic process, socialization, and facilitation of expression of feelings as group goals.

Problem of Noncompliance

1. Noncompliance is a major problem in administering drugs to psychiatric patients. It is the most important reason for recurring symptoms and rehospitalizations.
2. Dysphoric responses to the medication (*i.e.*, feelings of being in space, slowed down, confused, fearful, and nervous) contribute to noncompliance with antipsychotics.
3. The sedative and anticholinergic effects (*i.e.*, constipation, dry mouth, blurred vision, urinary retention, and palpitations) affect the compliance of patients on antidepressants.
4. Patients may prefer the "highs" to the side effects of lithium and choose to discontinue the medicine.
5. Use of long-acting antipsychotic is advised as one answer to the problem of compliance. Prolixin Decanoate lasts 3 to 4 weeks. Prolixin Enanthate lasts 10 days to 2 weeks.
6. Administration of psychotropics in a bedtime dose assists the patient in dealing with some bothersome side effects and in remembering to take it.

7. Education of patients about the effects of the drug is helpful in dealing with noncompliance.
8. The importance of the doctor–patient and/or nurse–patient relationship in promoting compliance is vital.

Antipsychotic Neuroleptic Drugs

Antipsychotic drugs are effective in treatment of psychoses (*i.e.*, schizophrenias); bipolar disorder, manic phase; neuroses; withdrawal of alcohol; nausea and vomiting. All the antipsychotic drugs listed in Table 5-1 are equally effective in relieving psychosis. They differ mostly in the type of side effects produced. Haldol is considered to be the most potent. Lithium and Tegretol also have antipsychotic effects and will be discussed in separate section.

TABLE 5-1. **Antipsychotic Neuroleptic Drugs**

Major Groups	Representative Drugs		Daily PO Doses (Range)
	Generic Name	*Trade Name*	
Phenothiazines			
Aliphatics	Chlorpromazine*	Thorazine*	300–2000 mg
	Triflupromazine	Vesprin	100–300 mg
	Promazine	Sparine	40–1000 mg
Piperazines	Acetophenazine	Tindal	60–600 mg
	Butaperazine	Repoise	15–100 mg
	Carphenazine	Proketazine	20–100 mg
	Fluphenazine	Prolixin	
	hydrochloride	hydrochloride	2.5–30 mg
	decanoate	decanoate	12.5–100 mg $\overline{q}$ 1–4 wks
	enanthate	enanthate	12.5–100 mg $\overline{q}$ 1–2 wks
	Perphenazine	Trilafon	8–64 mg
	Prochlorperazine	Compazine	
	Trifluoperazine*	Stelazine*	6–60 mg
Piperidines	Mesoridazine*	Serentil*	75–400 mg
	Piperacetazine	Quide	20–200 mg
	Thioridazine*	Mellaril*	200–800 mg
Nonphenothiazines			
Butyrophenones	Haloperidol*	Haldol*	6–100 mg
	Droperidol	Inapsine	2.5–5 mg
Thioxanthenes	Thiothixene*	Navane*	6–60 mg
Dibenzoxazepines	Loxapine*	Loxitane,* Daxolin	60–250 mg
Indolics	Molindone*	Lidone Moban*	50–400 mg

* Major drug(s) of the group.

Side Effects and Major Groups

1. *Sedative and hypotensive effects*
   a. If the drug has a sedative effect, it also decreases blood pressure.
   b. Aliphatics—*Thorazine* reduces blood pressure the most and has the greatest sedative effect.
   c. Piperazines and nonphenothiazines—*Stelazine* does not cause sedation and does not lower blood pressure.
   d. Piperidines—*Mellaril, Serentil* have almost the same sedative effect as Thorazine and a moderate effect in decreasing the blood pressure.
2. *Anticholinergic effects*—Dry mouth, constipation, urinary retention, blurred vision, tachycardia, confusion, memory loss, and interference with ability to think clearly.*
   a. Aliphatics—*Thorazine* has moderate anticholinergic effect.
   b. Piperazine and nonphenothiazines—*Stelazine* has least anticholinergic effect.
   c. Piperidines—*Mellaril, Serentil* have greatest anticholinergic effects.
3. *Extrapyramidal effects (EPS)*—Pseudoparkinsonism, akinesia, akathisia, dystonia.
   a. Aliphatics—*Thorazine* has moderate extrapyramidal effects.
   b. Piperazines and nonphenothiazines—Stelazine has greatest extrapyramidal effect.
   c. Piperidines—*Mellaril, Serantil* have the least extrapyramidal effects.

Mechanism of Action

Probably the blocking of dopamine receptors causes a decrease in psychotic symptoms. The drug is metabolized in the liver and excreted by the kidney.

Drug Effectiveness

1. Goal is to maintain the antipsychotic effect on the lowest possible dose.
2. Initial therapy begins with divided doses so that the patient can be monitored.
3. Rapid neuroleptization for acutely ill psychotic patients may be instituted.
   a. Give patient intramuscular haloperidol—for example, 5 mg every 30 to 60 minutes over a 2- to 6-hour period. IM haloperidol has peak serum levels in 20 to 40 minutes.
   b. Monitor blood pressure for hypotension before each dose; withhold dose if BP is 90 or below systolic.
   c. Monitor sleep state to achieve a 6- to 7-hour period.
   d. Monitor for dystonia occurring 1 hour to 48 hours after beginning of treatment and treat with antiparkinsonism drug.
   e. Monitor patient for decrease in danger to himself and others.

---

* Antiparkinsonism drugs have anticholinergic effects. Therefore, the treatment of EPS with antiparkinsonism drugs will cause additional anticholinergic effects if the antipsychotic drug has moderate anticholinergic effects. The patient would experience even more constipation, dryer mouth, more urinary retention, and so forth.

4. Dosage may be divided throughout the day or be given at bedtime.
   a. Preferably it should be given at bedtime because its sedative effect assists in establishing normal sleep pattern.
   b. Better compliance is achieved with bedtime dose.
   c. There are fewer extrapyramidal/anticholinergic effects experienced by the patient.
5. Drug holidays of 1 to 3 days, when no drugs are administered, may be given when patient is on long-term use.
6. Trial withdrawals are recommended every 6 months or year.
7. Excretion of drugs from body occurs slowly. May be present in body for weeks after last dose. Recurring symptoms of mental illness may not be experienced for weeks or months, reinforcing patient's belief that no medication is needed.
8. Antacid and diarrhea medications interfere with drug absorption; therefore, give antipsychotic 1 hour before or after the antacid or diarrhea drugs.
9. Recommended time periods for maintenance on drug.
   a. First psychotic episode: 6-month period.
   b. Second psychotic episode: 1-year period
   c. Third or later psychotic episode: indefinite period
10. When discontinuing the drug, the physician tapers the dosage because rapid withdrawal cause dyskinesia.

Responses to Treatment

1. Initially the patient is drowsy and cooperative within hours to a week.
2. The patient becomes more sociable and less withdrawn during next 2 months.
3. The thought disorder generally disappears in 6 weeks or more.
4. Improvement is generally noted in hallucinations, acute delusions, sleeping habits, appetite, tension, combativeness, hostility, negativism, and dress.
5. Lack of response to treatment is frequently related to failure to take the drug.
6. Polypharmacy or use of more than 1 phenothiazine is not necessary nor recommended.
7. Geriatric patients respond to lower dosages and may have hypotension because of the prolonged half-life of the drug in people over 55 years of age.

Side Effects

Side effects are treated with adjustments in kind and dosage of antipsychotic drug, with anticholinergic/antiparkinsonisn drugs, and other medical tests and treatments as indicated.

A. Drowsiness

1. Drowsiness is present especially when drug is started.
2. Tolerance will develop in about 2 weeks.
3. Activities such as driving a car or repairing delicate equipment should be avoided because alertness and muscular coordination are needed.

4. Medication may be given before bedtime, thereby decreasing the awareness of this side effect.

B. Orthostatic hypotension
1. Occurs more often after IM injections.
2. Symptoms are dizziness and weakness.
3. BP is below normal; systolic BP 90 or below is dangerous
4. Patient should change positions slowly.
5. BP should be monitored while patient is standing and sitting if symptoms of hypotension exist.
6. Dosage may be adjusted or medication changed or discontinued if symptoms persist.
7. Lower head and raise feet slightly to raise BP.
8. *Danger:* falling and sustaining injury.

C. Extrapyramidal symptoms (EPS)
1. *Dystonia*—Spasms of muscles of face, neck, back, eye, arms and legs.
    a. *Oculogyric crisis*—Fixed upward gaze from spasm of the oculomotor muscles.
    b. *Torticollis*—Pulling of head to the side from spasms of cervical muscles.
    c. *Opisthotonus*—Hyperextension of back from spasms of back muscles.
2. *Akathesia*—Continuous motor restlessness.
3. *Pseudoparkinsonism*—Shuffling gait; masklike facial expression; drooling; tremor; rigidity; and akinesia, which is experienced as weakness and fatigue.
4. *Akinesia*—Lack of body movement, especially in arms; frequently not treated because it is not striking and patient seldom complains.
5. EPS may occur 2 hours following an antipsychotic drug.
6. Dosage may be adjusted or medication changed, or an antiparkinsonism drug may be given for the first weeks of drug therapy.
7. Relief from severe reactions should occur 15 to 30 minutes after IM dose of antiparkinsonism drug.

D. Tardive dyskinesia
Serious because there is no known effective treatment.
1. Early symptoms are wormlike movements of tongue and frequent blinking.
2. Other symptoms include involuntary movements of tongue, lips, and jaw; chorea; tics; athetosis; and dystonia.
3. Usually occurs after 10 to 15 years of treatment; may occur as early as after 3 months of treatment.
4. There is a relationship between the use of neuroleptic drugs and tardive dyskinesia.
    a. Advantages and disadvantages of neuroleptics need to be discussed with patient.
    b. It is suggested that documentation of agreement to take neuroleptics with full knowledge of the possible effects of tardive dyskinesia be done.

5. Treatment
   a. Consists of lowering the dose of neuroleptics, or change of medication, or withdrawal of medication
   b. No treatment is uniformly effective.
   c. Lithium or diazepam may be used.
6. Evaluation of neuroleptic medication every 6 months, which includes a trial reduction of the medication, is recommended.

E. Convulsive seizures
1. May occur because the threshold is lowered.
2. Antipsychotic dosage is lowered and perhaps an anticonvulsant added.

F. Autonomic nervous system effects
1. Effects are caused by a blocking of cholinergic receptors
2. Symptoms are tachycardia, dry mouth, constipation, blurred vision, paralytic ileus, bladder paralysis.
3. Treatment
   a. Lowering of dosage aids in relief of these symptoms.
   b. Frequent fluids, sugarless gum, candy, or lozenges are used to relieve dry mouth.
   c. Diet, fluids, and laxatives may relieve constipation.

G. Allergic or toxic effects (rare and serious)
1. Agranulocytosis
   a. Symptoms are rapid onset of sore throat and fever.
   b. Occurs in first 3 to 8 weeks of treatment.
   c. Treatment: Stop the drug immediately, use reverse isolation technique, and administer antibiotics.
   d. Mortality rate is 30%.
2. Oral monoliasis
3. Dermatitis
4. Jaundice
   a. Note color of stool (pale) and urine (dark).
   b. Treatment consists of discontinuing medication.

H. Endocrine or metabolic effects
1. Weight gain; indicates need for exercise and dietary adjustments.
2. Menstrual irregularities and excessive secretion of mammary gland in females; indicates need for dosage adjustment.
3. Decreased libido, impotence, impaired ejaculation in males. Patient may be too embarrassed to report. Treatment generally consists of changing the antipsychotic drug and lowering the dosage.
4. Decreased thermoregulatory ability
   a. Complaints of being too hot or too cold.
   b. Care should be taken in use of ice bag or hot water bottle.

I. Miscellaneous

1. Toxic retinopathy
   a. Symptoms are disturbed color vision, especially brown tones; decreased visual acuity.
   b. Is believed to be related to Mellaril dosage of over 1200 mg daily.
2. Phenothiazine lens disease
   a. Does not affect visual acuity. Is partially reversible.
   b. Recommended eye examination every 3 to 12 months and minimal dosage of medication.
3. Photoxicity
   a. Excessive sun exposure may result in burn or rash.
   b. Sunscreens and adequate clothing are recommended.
4. Glycosuria—Carbohydrate metabolism may be affected. Medication and diet adjustments may be indicated; diabetic patient needs to have symptom explored and treated.
5. Urine may burn pinkish to red; effect is harmless.
6. Purplish-gray skin tone may occur after long-term use of drug.

Contraindications

Comatose states, glaucoma, prostatic hyperplasia, acute myocardial infarction are contraindications to use of these drugs.

Cautions

1. No birth defects have been caused by these drugs, but side effects (*e.g.*, muscle cramps) have been reported in infants.
2. Breast milk may contain the drug because some drugs pass into the milk, but this is considered safe.
3. Inhibition of growth hormone in children is possible after long-term therapy; therefore, careful evaluation of child's growth pattern is important.
4. Some physicians may advise discontinuance of drug prior to surgery.

Drug Interactions

1. Alcohol, barbiturates, and other CNS drugs—Sedation and hypotension are potentiated when antipsychotics and alcohol, barbiturates, and other CNS drugs are combined.
2. Antiparkinsonism and tricyclics—Dry mouth, postural hypotension, urinary retention, and constipation are increased when antipsychotics and antiparkinsonism drugs or tricyclics are combined.

Withdrawal Syndrome

1. Sweating, diarrhea, nausea, vomiting, insomnia, restlessness, tremor.
2. May be associated with cholinergic rebound, CNS stimulation, emerging tardive dyskinesia, and great sensitivity to stress.

Overdose

1. Symptoms are increased sedation, hypotension, and extrapyramidal signs.
2. Treatment includes gastric lavage, antiparkinsonism drugs, IV fluids, and norepinephrine for decreased blood pressure.

Nursing Alert: Neosynephrine may be administered to raise the BP when it is dangerously low. Epinephrine is not used because this will cause further lowering of blood pressure.

Rare Life-Threatening Side Effects

1. Neuroleptic malignant syndrome (NMS)
   a. Symptoms are hyperpyrexia, severe muscular rigidity, and autonomic nervous system dysfunction (*i.e.,* hypertension, hypotension, diaphoresis, and altered states of consciousness).
   b. Predisposing factors are dehydration, prolonged agitation, and prior treatment with lithium combined with current lithium treatment with high-dose, high-potency neuroleptic.
   c. Although some patients recover completely, mortality is reported at 20% and is related to respiratory failure, renal failure, and cardiovascular collapse.
   d. Treatment
      (1) Discontinuance of antipsychotics
      (2) Supportive care to lower temperature, prevent infection, and relax muscles
      (3) Diuresis
2. Catatonia
   a. Symptoms are similar to those of catatonic stupor (*i.e.,* waxy flexibility, withdrawal, regression, muscular rigidity). Most important symptom is appearance of symptoms shortly following administration of antipsychotic.
   b. *Note:* Increase in symptoms may lead to increase of antipsychotic drug with consequent deterioration of condition of patient.
   c. Treatment consists of cessation of antipsychotic medication and institution of supportive measures.
3. Laryngeal spasm—Respiratory distress is treated with IM diphenhydramine (Benadryl) or IV benztropine (Cogentin).
4. Hyperpyrexia
   a. Caused by suppression of hypothalamus by neuroleptics, heat, humidity, and exercise.
   b. Symptoms are severe hyperpyrexia, lack of sweating, and dysfunctional central nervous system.
   c. Treatment consists of following treatment principles for heat stroke with techniques to lower body temperature and to maintain respiratory and cardiovascular systems.

Antidepressant Drugs

Antidepressant drugs (Table 5-2) are used to treat affective disorders.

Mechanism of Action

These drugs act by increasing norepinephrine and serotonin, which are metabolized in the liver and excreted in the urine.

TABLE 5-2. **Antidepressant Drugs**

Major Groups	Representative Drugs		Daily PO Doses (Range)
	Generic Name	*Trade Name*	
Tricyclic Antidepressants	Amitriptyline	Elavil	75–300 mg
	Desipramine	Norpramin	100–300 mg
	Imipramine	Tofranil	100–300 mg
	Nortriptyline	Aventyl	75–150 mg
	Protriptyline	Vivactil	15–60 mg
	Doxepin	Sinequan	75–300 mg
Tetracyclic Antidepressants	Maprotiline	Ludiomil	75–300 mg
Monoamine Oxidase Inhibitors	Isocarboxazid	Marplan	
	Phenelzine	Nardil	
	Tranylcypromine	Parnate	
Miscellaneous	Trazodone	Desyrel	200–600 mg

Drug Effectiveness

1. Dosage may be divided throughout the day, but preferably the total dose is given at bedtime because of the sedative effects.
2. A minimum dose is initially given and then gradually increased.
3. There may be no immediate changes in mood because there is a lag of 5 to 21 days.
4. Therapeutic effect may take 4 to 6 weeks to achieve.
5. Psychomotor activity increases before patient states he actually feels better.
6. Medication may be continued for 6 months after patient is free from depression.

Response to Treatment

1. Drowsiness may occur and subside after initial period. Patient is warned about driving car or operating other equipment that requires alertness.
2. Initially, hypotension may be experienced. Advise patient that he may feel faint and to change positions slowly.
3. Discontinuance of therapy is done by tapering the dosage. Otherwise, withdrawal symptoms are experienced.
4. Geriatric patients are more sensitive to the drug and its side effects, especially hypotension. Lower dosages are indicated. *Danger:* The patient may fall when under the influence of these drugs.

Side Effects

Anticholinergic effects from tricyclics and monamine oxidase inhibitors are generally mild (*i.e.,* dry mouth, constipation, blurred vision, tachycardia, nausea, edema, hypotension, and urinary retention). These side effects are treated by adjustment of dosage and supportive measures. (See discussion of antipsychotic drugs.)

A. Tricyclics

1. Allergic reactions may occur (*i.e.,* skin rash and jaundice).
2. Cardiovascular effects—Major symptom is tachycardia, which is treated by careful monitoring or change of medication, or both.
3. Tremor is experienced.
4. Blood dyscrasias develop during long-term therapy. Bone marrow is depressed, causing symptoms of fever, sore throat, and aching. Treatment consists of cessation of the drug.

B. Monoamine oxidase inhibitors

1. Liver damage; rare but fatal.
2. Precipitation of manic episode
3. Hypertensive crises
   a. Occurs 30 minutes to 24 hours after eating foods containing tyramine (cheese, wine, beer, sour cream, chocolate, liver, pickled herring, raisins, bananas, avocados, soy sauce, fava beans).
   b. Symptoms are severe headache, palpitation, neck stiffness, nausea, vomiting, increased BP, chest pain, collapse.
   c. Treatment consists of discontinuance of monoamine oxidase inhibitors and administration of Regitine to lower the blood pressure.

Contraindications

Glaucoma, agitated states, urinary retention, cardiac disorders, seizure disorders.

Drug Interactions

1. Many interactions are reported; therefore, refer to current list of drug interactions or pharmacist when other drugs are being given.
2. Alcohol—Sedative and hypotensive effects are potentiated when antidepressants are given with alcohol.
3. Anticholinergics and antidepressants given together cause an additive effect.
4. Monoamines and antidepressants given together cause central adrenergic reaction; can be fatal.

Cautions

1. Drugs should be discontinued prior to surgery.
2. Psychotic state may be produced in patients with chronic brain syndrome, bipolar disorder, or schizophrenia. Treatment consists of discontinuance of drug.

> *Nursing Alert: Suicide potential is greater as patient begins to feel more energetic and depression lifts as a result of drug treatment and other therapies.*

Withdrawal

Symptoms of nausea and headache are experienced if drug is discontinued or stopped suddenly.

Overdose

1. Tricyclics
   a. Symptoms are cardiac arrhythmia, convulsion, low blood pressure, respiratory depression, mydriasis, and delirium.
   b. Treatment consists of lavage, supportive treatment to maintain respiratory function and adequate blood pressure, and control of seizures and cardiac arrhythmia.
2. Monamine oxidase inhibitors
   a. Symptoms are coma, increased respirations, tachycardia, and hyperthermia. Note that there is a 1- to 6-hour lag before serious symptoms appear.
   b. Treatment is symptomatic; dialysis also can be used.

Antimanic Drugs

Lithium Salts

Lithium (Table 5-3) is used to treat bipolar disorder, manic phase, and periodic impulsive aggressiveness.

Mechanism of Action

Lithium is believed to inhibit availability of norepinephrine to receptors and change sodium transport. It is excreted rapidly by the kidneys.

Drug Effectiveness

1. Drug is given 2 to 3 times a day because of its rapid excretion from body; is given at mealtime to those susceptible to nausea.
2. Toxic and therapeutic blood lithium levels are close to each other and require careful monitoring.
   a. In maintenance states, the therapeutic range is 0.6 to 0.9 mEq, measured every 4 to 6 weeks.
   b. Lithium blood levels are drawn at least 8 to 12 hours after last dose.
3. Adequate kidney function and sodium balance and hydration are essential to lithium excretion.
   a. The sodium balance is affected by low-salt diets, fad diets, and diet pills that lead to reduction in food and fluids. Conversely, foods and drugs

TABLE 5-3. **Antimanic Drugs**

| Major Groups | Representative Drugs | | Daily PO Doses (Range) |
	Generic Name	*Trade Name*	
Lithium	Lithium salts	Lithane Lithonate Eskalith	300–2400 mg

high in sodium may be used excessively, effecting change in sodium levels (*e.g.,* diet sodas, antacids and corned beef).
   b. Patient is encouraged to consume 2 to 3 quarts of fluids per day because urination may be more frequent as the kidney excretes lithium.
   c. Coffee, tea and colas in large amounts (over 10 cups per day) also may promote the excretion of lithium because of the diuretic effect of the caffeine in these drinks. Caffeine also acts as stimulant when stabilization of mood is wanted.
   d. During strenuous exercise, maintenance of fluid intake is important for preventing dehydration; lithium toxicity risk is not increased.

Responses to Treatment

1. Drowsiness may be experienced, so extra precautions need to be taken if patient is handling mechanical equipment and driving.
2. Initially, the patient will experience side effects, which may subside after 1 to 2 weeks. They are
   a. Nausea, vomiting, diarrhea, thirst, and weight loss.
   b. Hand tremors and muscle weakness.
   c. Polyuria (may wet the bed at night).
   d. Swelling in hands and feet.
   e. Decrease in sexual functioning.
3. There is a 5- to 10-day lag in the therapeutic effect.
4. Leveling of mood swings, improved sleep pattern, decrease in agitation, less grandiosity, less hyperactivity, and improved judgment will occur.
5. Geriatric patients require less lithium, probably because the kidneys of people in this age group have decreased ability to excrete it.
6. There may be some T-wave changes on ECG. Leukocytosis also may develop.

Side Effects Related to Long-Term Use

1. Hand tremor—Treatment consists of decreasing lithium level.
2. Polyuria and polydipsia
   a. Caused by blockage of antidiuretic hormone (ADH), resulting in decreased ability to concentrate urine.
   b. Symptoms are polyuria, thirst, weight gain, and nocturia. Not considered reason to discontinue lithium.
   c. There is no proven treatment.
3. Approach to weight gain includes dietary instruction about avoiding high-calorie drinks and having a sufficient amount of sodium intake.
4. GI distress, pain, and diarrhea
   a. Caused by presence of unabsorbed lithium irritating the large intestine.
   b. Treated by changing type of lithium and by having smaller, frequent doses.
5. Depressed thyroid function
   a. There is an asymptomatic enlargement of thyroid after long-term use of lithium.

b. Symptoms of hypothyroidism are tiredness, coldness in extremities, headache, myxedema, decreased T_3 and T_4, and increased TSH.

c. Treated by discontinuance of lithium and thyroid medications.

6. Acne and psoriasis

Contraindications

Cardiovascular disease, renal disorders, epilepsy, dehydration.

Cautions

1. Lithium and haloperidol combinations or other combinations of neuroleptics with lithium may be associated with kidney problem; therefore, careful monitoring is required.
2. During pregnancy, there is increased danger of toxicity.
3. With fever, sweating, and/or diarrhea, the amount of lithium required will be less, and danger of toxicity will be greater.
4. Breast-feeding is not recommended because the infant may develop toxicity.
5. Lithium may be discontinued prior to surgery and restarted the following day.

Drug Interactions

1. Antipsychotic drugs—Nausea, which is a sign of lithium toxicity, may be decreased or blocked when antipsychotic drugs are given with lithium.
2. Diuretics or steroids—Electrolyte imbalance may be possible when lithium and diuretics or steroid preparations are given together.

Toxicity

1. Caused by kidney disease, severe dehydration, or too much lithium.
2. Early symptoms are muscle weakness, diarrhea, vomiting, lack of coordination, tremor, and slurred speech.
3. Symptoms at high levels (approximately 2 mEq/hour) are ataxia, coarse tremors, blurred vision, faintness, tinnitus, large urinary output, drowsiness, confusion, and lack of memory.
4. Symptoms of an overdose are vomiting, increasing weakness, lack of coordination, athetotic movements, hypotension, seizures, coma, and cardiac arrhythmias.
5. Treatment consists of discontinuance of drug, administration of fluids, correction of fluid and electrolyte imbalance, and protection of kidney function.
6. Response to treatment is monitored by observation of daily electrolytes, hematocrit, lithium level, and body weight.

Rare Conditions

1. Nephrotoxicity may be related to long-term use of lithium, lithium blood levels, adequacy of fluids with body, and concurrent use of psychotic drugs.
2. Lithium-induced organic brain syndrome. Symptoms are confusion, disorientation, ataxia, slurred speech, low to moderate lithium level, absence

of nausea, vomiting, and diarrhea. Treatment consists of discontinuance of lithium.

Carbamazepine (Tegretol)

Tegretol is used as an alternative to lithium in the treatment of bipolar disorder; it is a known treatment for seizure disorder.

Mechanism of action

Unknown. Drug is metabolized in the liver.

Side Effects

1. Drowsiness and dizziness—Advise patient to use caution when handling machinery.
2. Nausea and vomiting.
3. Anemia due to depression of bone marrow—Recommend periodic blood studies.

Contraindications

Glaucoma

Drug interactions

1. Doxycycline, a tetracycline—Antimicrobial action is decreased when used with Tegretol.
2. Anticoagulants. Tegretol affects the metabolism of oral anticoagulants; therefore, dosage requirements need careful monitoring.

Antianxiety Drugs

Antianxiety drugs (minor tranquilizers, anxiolytics relaxants; Table 5-4) are used to treat psychoneurotic disorders, anxiety disorders, and alcohol detoxification and preoperatively to reduce anxiety.

TABLE 5-4. **Antianxiety Drugs**

| Major Classes | Representative Drugs | | Daily PO Doses (Range) |
	Generic Name	Trade Name	
Propanediols	Meprobamate	Equanil Miltown	800–1000 mg
	Tybamate	Solacen Tybatran	500–1000 mg
Benzodiazepines	Clorazepate	Tranxene	15–60 mg
	Chlordiazepoxide	Librium	25–80 mg
	Diazeparn	Valium	10–40 mg
	Oxazepam	Serax	10–60 mg
	Flurazepam	Dalmane	15–30 mg
Diphenylmethanes	Diphenhydra-mine	Benadryl	25–200 mg
	Hydroxyzine	Atarax Vistaril	50–400 mg

Mechanism of Action

Affects limbic system through the neurotransmitter GABA. It is metabolized in the liver and excreted in the urine.

Drug Effectiveness

1. Drug therapy is generally short-term to relieve anxiety in neuroses and personality disorders.
2. Within 30 to 60 minutes after taking the drug orally, the patient experiences some calming and sedative effects. Maximum effect of the drug is generally experienced in a couple of days.
3. Tolerance to drugs may develop in 3 to 4 weeks, or in even less time.
4. Geriatric patients require lower dosages.

Side Effects

1. Drowsiness—Caution patient against use of machinery that requires quick action, such as car.
2. Faintness and dizziness—May result from hypotension. Advise patient to change position slowly.
3. There is low incidence of autonomic and extrapyramidal effects.

Contraindications

Severe depression, glaucoma, psychoses.

Drug Interactions

1. Alcohol, barbiturates, and other CNS depressants—Sedative effects potentiated when antianxiety drugs are given with these drugs.
2. Antidepressants: Sedation, dry mouth, blurred vision, rapid pulse, flushed face, and urinary retention effects are potentiated when antianxiety drugs are given with antidepressants.
3. Antihypertensive effects are potentiated when Valium is given with diuretics and antihypertensive drugs.

Cautions

1. Physical dependence may occur.
2. Potential for misuse is great.
3. Suicide potential may be greater as anxiety is reduced.
4. Faintness, slurred speech, and ataxia may indicate that the patient is taking more than prescribed.
5. Breast milk will contain the drugs if mother is taking them. Safety during pregnancy has not been proved.

Withdrawal

Symptoms include nervousness, weakness, restlessness, vomiting, sweating, muscle cramps, anorexia, and convulsions.

Overdose

1. Symptoms are coma, confusion, diminished reflexes.
2. Treatment consists of lavage and maintenance of respiratory and cardiovascular functions.

TABLE 5-5. **Anticholinergic/Antiparkinsonism Drugs**

| Major Classes | Representative Drugs | | Daily PO Doses (Range) |
	Generic Name	*Trade Name*	
Anticholinergics	Trihexyphenidyl	Artane	2–15 mg
	Benztropine	Cogentin	0.5–6 mg
	Biperiden	Akineton	2–8 mg
	Procyclidine	Kemadrin	2–20 mg
Miscellaneous	Diphenhydramine hydrochloride	Benadryl	25–200 mg

Anticholinergic/Antiparkinsonism Drugs

Anticholinergic/antiparkinsonism drugs (Table 5-5) are used to alleviate the side effects of antipsychotics.

Mechanism of Action

Reduction of cholinergic activity.

Drug Effectiveness

1. Drug therapy is given in divided doses to treat drug-induced extrapyramidal symptoms.
2. Controversy over prophylactic use exists.
3. Drug may be discontinued after 1 to 3 months, with only few patients requiring resumption of medication, even though they are still taking an antipyschotic.
4. Phenothiazines should be discontinued before antiparkinsonism drug is stopped because of the slow excretion of phenothiazines.

Side Effects

Dry mouth, blurred vision, constipation, drowsiness, nausea, nervousness, and urinary retention. (See discussion of side effects of antipsychotics.)

Contraindications

Glaucoma, prostatic hyperplasia.

Drug Interactions

1. Blurred vision, dry mouth, constipation, and other anticholinergic actions are additive when tricyclic antidepressants or antipsychotics are given with antiparkinsonism drugs.
2. Neurological symptoms are potentiated when monamine oxidase inhibitors are given with antiparkinsonism drugs.

PROTECTIVE INTERVENTIONS
Observation for Suicide Prevention

Observation for suicide prevention is a procedure in which the nurse–patient relationship is continuously used to prevent suicide.

Purpose

1. To protect patient from self-injury or death.
2. To increase patient's control of self-destructive impulses.
3. To provide opportunity to talk about the pain, feelings (especially the anger towards self and others, the hopelessness, the helplessness), and problems.

Nursing Interventions

1. Establish a relationship with the patient.
   a. Begin by explaining who you are and what you are going to do with and for him.
   b. Convey empathy for his feelings and view of life.
   c. Assist in describing the suicide attempt.
   d. Verbalize that patient's attempt to take his life is not "bad."
2. Stay with patient at arm's length at all times during waking hours.
3. Have patient sleep in area that facilitates constant observation. Distance of nurse from the patient may increase.
4. Discuss with patient the activities of the day, and plan for patient to attend as many activities as possible.
5. Make a verbal or written contract with patient not to harm self further.
6. Help patient contact a friend, spouse, parent, or other significant person.
7. Assess the suicide risk.
   a. Are suicidal ideas or wishes still present?
   b. Has the plan for suicide changed?
   c. How will others be affected?
   d. Is there danger for others as well as self?
   e. Is he viewing the act as the only way, or is he open to other views?
   f. Is the feeling of hopelessness present?
8. Discuss with team members daily the continuance of the procedure.

Activity Area Restriction

Room restriction is a method of limiting movement of the patient to a specific room. *Area restriction* is a method of limiting movement of the patient to a large room or rooms, such as a lounge or dayroom.

Purpose

1. To protect patient from self-injury or injury to others.
2. To assist patient in controlling impulses.
3. To provide time to think through current situation.

Nursing Interventions

1. Explain procedure, including purpose and time period of the restriction.
2. Provide support to stay within area.
3. Give patient feedback about inappropriate behavior immediately and help him modify the behavior.

Seclusion

Seclusion is placement of the patient in a protected room with a locked door.

Nursing Alert: Basic to the use of this controversial method of treatment is the assumption that other interventions were tried and did not succeed in reducing the behavior. Physician's order is needed.

Purpose

1. To provide protection from self-injury and injury to others only when the danger is clearly recognized.
2. To prevent gross damage or disruption to the environment.
3. To re-establish control of aggressive impulses and a more neutral, if not positive, relationship with environment.

Nursing Interventions

1. Provide protected room that generally includes no furnishings, soundly constructed walls and floor, door that cannot be opened from the inside, mattress and blankets that cannot be destroyed easily, protected window, light fixture, and ventilation equipment.
2. Obtain additional staff to escort patient into seclusion and later to escort patient to bathroom, to provide opportunity to smoke, to give food at meal times, to take vital signs, and so on. Give clear, brief explanations.
3. State calmly and concisely the reason for the treatment, when the next meal is expected, the safety of the room, when staff will check on him, how to ask for additional help, approximate length of treatment, and behaviors necessary for release.
4. Have patient remove clothing and jewelry, and provide him with gown or shorts and tee shirt. Clothing may have to be completely absent if patient is actively attempting to kill himself. Otherwise, patient should have one layer of clothing to maintain some sense of privacy, respect, and warmth.
5. Tell patient what is happening to his personal belongings. List items removed from patient and place in locked area.
6. Provide urinal or explain to patient how to let staff know that he needs to go to the bathroom. Offer bathroom facilities every 2 to 3 hours.
7. Offer fluids frequently or leave container in room.
8. Make frequent and regular checks of patient (every 15 minutes is suggested; more frequent checks may be necessary if patient is very agitated).
9. Verbally acknowledge your presence to the patient at each check. For example, call his name, give time of day. Elicit his thoughts and feelings.
10. Serve food in paper containers and remove uneaten portions promptly. Assist patient in eating if necessary.
11. Check vital signs or at least blood pressure before administering antipsychotic medication.
12. Continue to give prn medications prescribed for agitation.
13. Investigate by entering room and talking to or inspecting patient; determine whether patient remains in one position for prolonged period or whether unusual noise or activity is noted.
14. Enter room hourly to check temperature, cleanliness, and safety of environment. Arrange for daily cleaning of room area.

15. Provide for daily bath and cleaning of teeth and other grooming needs as needed and tolerated.
16. Contract with patient to maintain control of behavior.
17. Begin some teaching of how to control his behavior by
    a. Stating that violence is not acceptable and will be controlled.
    b. Teaching the STOP/LOOK/LISTEN technique.
    c. Teaching a relaxation method (*e.g.,* imagining a quiet, safe place where he has all his wants met).
18. Assess the patient's need for continued treatment:
    a. How does he respond to nurse's voice, offering of explanations, giving of treatments?
    b. What behavior does he exhibit when assisted in bathing or toileting or when given meals?
    c. Can he wait a moment for things he wants, or is he very demanding or confused?
    d. Is he responding to imaginary voices?
    e. How long does he remain oriented?
    f. Are there changes in level of consciousness, is the patient more disoriented, is there more impairment of memory?
    g. What evidence is there that his paranoid thinking is continuing?
19. Provide opportunity to discuss staff's beliefs and feelings about seclusion of patient and also what can be done to prevent its use in future.
20. Following seclusion treatment, discuss with patient reasons for it and what staff did for him.

Restraints

Handcuffs are two metal, ringlike devices connected by a short chain and locked around the wrists. *Wristlets* are wide, leather, padded cuffs secured with a leather strap and locking device. They can be attached to wrists or ankles of the patient and then secured to the waist or to a bed. *Limb and body holders* are special devices used to hold a body part in a bed or chair. *Sheet restraint* is a folded sheet placed over body part and fastened to a bed or chair that is out of the reach of the patient.

Purpose

1. To provide protection from injury to self and others.
2. To increase patient's control of self-destructive impulses.

Nursing Intervention

1. Explain reasons for application of restraint.
2. Provide continuous monitoring of patient's response to procedure.
3. Check skin areas for signs of irritation.
4. Assure some movement of body part.
5. Release restraints prn (at least every 2 hours is suggested) or to allow patient to eat and go to the bathroom.
6. Provide for limited activity.
7. Encourage recognition by patient that a time-out period or activity restriction is needed and can be requested at another time.

8. When all extremities are restrained
   a. Place patient on side or stomach. Change his position every 2 hours.
   b. Release restraints one at a time prn and at least every 2 hours to allow patient to eat or go to the bathroom. If patient's level of agitation does not permit an active exercise for limbs, then do passive range of motion again as patient's condition permits.
   c. Provide 1:1 special observation if patient is in four-point restraint.

Protective Interventions in Violent Situations

Nursing Interventions with Suggested Comments

A. Sequence I: Interventions using interpersonal techniques

1. Move other patients out of area.
   "Can you go into another room so Mr. X and I can work something out."
2. Allow increased distance between self and patient.
   "I'll stay here." (Said in calm, respectful manner.)
3. Obtain additional help.
   "Ms. X is calling for some assistance."
4. Identify your concern.
   "Something serious has happened to upset you so . . ."
5. Offer assistance; offer fluids, food, and so on.
   "I would like to help . . ."
6. Give positive reassurance to patient that he will be assisted in maintaining control and prevented from hurting self or others.
   "I do not want you to hurt anyone. I cannot allow that . . ."
7. Suggest alternatives to present behavior.
   "Can you put down the chair so I can talk with you a bit more easily?" or "Can we walk down to my office?" or "How about a shower?"
8. Actively request verbalization of problem.
   "What went on . . ."

B. Sequence II: Interventions using physical restraint

Interventions using interpersonal techniques may not be successful in helping the patient achieve more rational control of his behavior, and physical restraint may be indicated.

1. Obtain additional help. At least four persons are recommended.
2. Explain to patient what type of restraint will be used to help him achieve control of his behavior.
3. Use necessary method to remove patient from the area, to place patient in seclusion or restraints, or to immobilize him.*
   a. One staff member with head lock and a half nelson.
   b. Two staff members using lever restraint. Each person rotates patient's wrist outward, keeping patient's elbow straight, and, with other hand under patient's arm, grasps his partner's hand.

---

* To ensure full understanding of these holds, arrange to see videotapes and demonstrations and to practice.

    c. Two staff members using shoulder restraint. Each person grasps patient's wrist and shoulder and swings patient's straight arm backward and up keeping elbow joint up.

    d. Two staff members using straight-arm restraint. Each person rotates patient's wrist outward and places other arm over the patient's arm and under his elbow.

    e. Four staff members using one man on each extremity.

4. Use blanket or mattress to distract patient while others are achieving physical restraint.

C. Interventions using measures to protect self

1. Have confidence in own ability to manage based on skills in assessing, planning, and acting in violent situations.

2. Be aware of cues of increasing aggression (*e.g.,* grinding teeth, pacing, making fist, pounding, using threatening words, becoming more angry and/or suspicious, increasing voice volume and pressure, experiencing existing turmoil in the environment, having feelings of fear generated in the participant observer).

3. Move slowly from side to side, allowing distance from patient as you talk with him, standing to the side of the patient, and avoiding constant, direct eye contact to decrease intensity of interaction.

4. Use the left/right back stance to achieve greater stability and flexibility. Do not turn your back on the patient.

5. Observe eye movements of patient because he will look at what he plans to attack, and you will have a chance to take preventive action.

6. Use objects in environment, such as a chair, to protect self from a blow with an object.

7. Avoid blows from patient who is sitting or lying on floor by kneeling on floor with knee close to patient in a bent position, but not touching floor.

8. Keep arms bent and in front of body to protect chest and face from blows.

9. Be prepared to act. Think of an ingenious way to escape, such as placing self near exist.

10. Use counter-projective speech to help the paranoid patient focus less on you as you begin to interact.

    a. Remarks are directed "out there." For example, "Your relatives really did a number this time."

    b. Speak about the "others," significant persons with whom he is angry or upset.

    c. Convey a feeling about the "others" that is similar to the patient's feeling.

Seizure Management

> *Nursing Alert: Many psychotropic medications lower the seizure threshold, increasing the need for observation, protection, and instruction of the patient.*

Purpose

1. To provide patient with protection from self-injury.
2. To prevent recurring seizures.

Nursing Interventions

1. Check patient for adequate airway.
2. Place gag, towel, or handkerchief in patient's mouth.
3. Turn patient's head to side.
4. Support head and extremities with blanket and firm grasp.
5. Note type of movements and body part affected, size of pupils, state of consciousness, duration, incontinence, and behavior following attack.
6. Have staff stay with patient until he is conscious, then check his need for orientation.
7. Discuss seizure with patient and ascertain whether there was any aura. Identify plans to control future seizures.
8. Assist patient in recording his seizures.
9. Discuss anticonvulsive medication with patient, stressing regularity in taking it.

REFERENCE

1. Yalom I: The Theory and Practice of Group Psychotherapy. New York, Basic Books, 1975

6

Major Psychiatric Disorders

SELECTED MENTAL DISORDERS

The American Psychiatric Association's *Diagnostic and Statistical Manual of Mental Disorders*[1] presents a multiaxial system for mental disorders. There are five axes on which each individual is evaluated. The first represents the official diagnostic assessment.

Axis 1: Clinical syndrome—Conditions not attributable to a mental disorder that are a focus for treatment.

Axis 2: Personality disorders—Specific developmental disorders.

Axis 3: Physical disorders and conditions.

Axis 4: Severity of psychosocial stresses.

Axis 5: Highest level of adaptive functioning during past year.

Examples of a diagnostic evaluation of a patient:

Axis 1: Bipolar disorder, manic episode with psychotic features.

Axis 2: Borderline.

Axis 3: Arthritis.

Axis 4: None known.

Axis 5: Very good.

Disorders from the 17 major classes have been selected for discussion on the basis of prevalence in adults.

Nursing Responsibilities

1. A nursing diagnosis is made for the individual patient. It identifies the problems or potential problems on which the nurse will take independent action. Following the discussion of the disorder, a list of commonly associated nursing diagnoses is given.
2. Further assessment factors are implied in the description of the clinical features and the etiological factors of the mental disorders. The nurses would observe for the presence and absence of these signs and symptoms

and thus assist the doctor as well as the patient with the treatment of the disorder.
3. Nursing actions are implied in the treatment. For example, acting on the knowledge that a disorder requires symptom relief, the nurse would help relieve the symptoms.
4. Nursing actions, specifically teaching activities, are identified in the Health Teaching section. Further specific areas for teaching will become apparent as the nurse continues to assess an individual patient and family.

Organic Mental Disorders

Organic mental disorders represent a group of mental disorders that present a variety of symptoms, especially a disturbance of cognition.

Incidence

1. Delirium is common in general hospitals, with an estimated 5% to 15% of patients exhibiting symptoms.
2. Dementia impairs about 1,000,000 people; Alzheimer's disease is the most common type.
3. Organic mental disorders affect 3,000,000 people to some degree.
4. Diagnosis of organic mental disorders is difficult; overdiagnosis and underdiagnosis exist. Careful examination and testing are necessary to rule out another condition that requires treatment.

Etiology

A. Delirium

1. Vascular disorders
2. Metabolic changes
3. Growth impairments
4. Nutritional deficiencies
5. Trauma
6. Drugs
7. Poison
8. Infections
9. Tumors
10. Epilepsy

B. Dementia

1. Alzheimer's disease (51% of cases)
   a. Specific cause unknown. There are Alzheimer-type neuropathological brain changes noted at autopsy.
   b. Defective genes
   c. Immune system dysfunction
   d. Alterations in the synthesis and release of neurotransmitters or other abnormalities in the intraneuronal processes
   e. Viral infections
   f. Aluminum deposits in the brain
   g. Head injuries
2. Vascular disease

3. Normal-pressure hydrocephalus
4. Alcoholism
5. Multiple other causes: neurosyphilis, brain tumors, pernicious anemia, thyroid disease, liver failure, epilepsy, drug toxicity

Clinical Features

A. Delirium

Sudden onset of impairment of all cognitive functions.
1. *State of consciousness impairment*
    a. Mild—Indecisiveness, weakness, problems in judging time, difficulty paying attention and thinking logically, episodes of untidiness.
    b. Severe—Drowsiness, sleeping most of day, inability to comprehend requests, frequent sleeping by day and state of excitement at night.
2. *Psychomotor impairment*—Varies from mild slowing (little spontaneous movement, apathy) to inactivity to overactivity and noisiness.
3. *Thinking impairment*
    a. Early signs—Problems in presenting complex ideas, increase in importance of own internal world, loss of insight.
    b. More severe signs—Concreteness and disorganization, inability to determine whether one is inside or outside, sitting or standing; persecutory delusions; mixing of past and present experiences.
4. *Memory impairment*
    a. May at first be to time (*e.g.,* a missing of sequences of time or not realizing that so much time has passed).
    b. Later impairment related to place and person with confabulations and false memories.
5. *Perception impairment*
    a. Occurs in visual field especially.
    b. Ranges from a blurring to changing shapes to hallucinations.
6. *Emotional impairment*—Ranges from early depression to later apathy.

B. Dementia

A slow deterioration in cognitive functioning causing multiple changes.
1. Symptoms are the same, regardless of age at onset of illness. First sign is loss of recent memory with preservation of long-term memory.
2. Signs/symptoms of dementia become worse with increasing anxiety and fatigue; therefore, the patient is worse at night.
3. Some authors differentiate between types:
    a. DAT: dementia, Alzheimer's type (symptoms appear before patient is 65 years of age).
    b. SDAT: senile dementia, Alzheimer's type (symptoms appear after patient is 65 years of age).
4. Early signs
    a. Losing objects
    b. Mixing up appointments
    c. Not being aware of recent occurrences
    d. Making mistakes with money
    e. Being inefficient at work

    f. Not grasping important things

    g. Displaying poor social manners, social blunders (stealing, exposing self), bizarre behavior (putting food in washing machine)

    h. Tiring easily

    i. Having poverty of ideas (cliches and set phrases said repeatedly)

    j. Showing forgetfulness, irritability, anxiety

5. Middle signs

    a. Neglect of personal hygiene and disordered appearance

    b. Indifference, sloppy eating manners

    c. Incontinence

    d. Aimlessness

    e. No new thoughts, inflexible

    f. Paranoid ideation

    g. Speech broken and used to obtain food or other physical needs

    h. Disorientation, apathy

    i. Euphoria at times

    j. Increasingly flat in affect

6. Later signs

    a. Limitation of speech to few words, then to unintelligible speech and grunts

    b. Inability to walk, feed self, or to perform other motor skills

    c. Stupor, then coma

C. Organic delusional syndrome

A disorder with delusions related to an organic factor such as amphetamines, alcohol, and cocaine.

D. Organic affective syndrome

A disorder with mood disturbance related to organic factor, such as amphetamines and hallucinogens.

E. Organic disorders associated with circulatory disturbances

1. Lack of cellular oxygenation results in ischemia or infarction with localized (lacunae) or diffuse changes.

2. Transient cerebral ischemic attacks (TIA) are episodes of dysfunction lasting 5 to 15 minutes and are risk factors for cerebral infarction.

F. Senile dementia

A disorder of unknown cause characterized by severe impairment of intellectual functioning; if it occurs when person is under 65 years of age, it is called Alzheimer's disease.

G. Focal cerebral disorders

1. *Frontal lobe*—Person has changes of personality with overfamiliarity, talkativeness, excitement, joking, punning, tactlessness.

2. *Parietal lobe*—Person has variety of cognitive disturbances.

3. *Temporal lobe*—Person has disturbance of intellectual functioning asso-

ciated with emotional instability and aggressive misconduct; epileptic phenomena.
4. *Occipital lobe*—Person has visual field effects.
5. *Corpus callosum*—Person has rapid intellectual deterioration.
6. *Diencephalon and brain stem*—Person has recent short-term memory loss and hypersomnia.

H. Organic mental disorders induced by drugs or poisons
1. *Intoxication*
   a. Generally includes changes in perception, attention, thinking, wakefulness, judgment, emotional control, and psychomotor behavior.
   b. The changes are directly related to the ingestion of specific substances.
   c. Most symptoms are related to decrease in level of consciousness, interfering with sensory input.
2. *Withdrawal*
   a. Generally includes anxiety, restlessness, insomnia, irritability, impaired attention, GI symptoms, weakness, desire for drug, sleep-pattern disturbances, convulsions.
   b. The symptoms are related to the ingestion of the specific substance.
3. *Sedatives and hypnotics* are associated with half of the cases of disorders induced by drugs or poisons.

Treatment

A. Delirium

Treatment of delirium is focused on elimination of physical cause; symptom relief; prevention of complications, especially injuries from falling; nutritional supplements; psychotropics to assist in agitation; and environmental management.

B. Dementia
1. Treatment of dementia is also directed towards elimination of any physical cause; however, in the majority of cases there is no specific treatment.
2. Other conditions affecting the elderly and the progression of dementia are: loss of loved ones, own pending death, lack of sufficient funds, malnutrition, over medication, aging process. The effect of these conditions needs to be carefully evaluated.
3. Depression is common in elderly persons and may be misdiagnosed as dementia; 25% of all suicides occur in that age group.
4. Other medical conditions are frequently present and are being treated with drugs that effect dementia or cause similar symptoms or both. These conditions include hypertension, arthritis, diabetes, hormone imbalance, and inflammation of arteries.
5. Treatment includes
   a. Continuous assessment of causes of symptoms and treatment as indicated.
   b. Group and/or individual psychotherapy with focus on management of

anxiety, loss, impending death, reality orientation, and changes in life-style.

   c. Neuroleptics or antidepressants are used to decrease agitation. They are used with extreme caution because of side effects that may lead to falls that result in injuries, particularly hip fractures.

   d. Metabolic enhancers (*i.e.,* lecithin, physostigmine).

   e. Drugs to improve circulation and neurotransmitter action.

   f. Environmental interventions to promote safety and security.

   g. Use of day treatment centers, in-patient services for further diagnoses, visiting nurse services, and nursing care homes.

   h. Family assessment and interventions for the grief reactions experienced. Stages of the reaction are similar to the grief response.

C. Disorder induced by drugs or poisons

Treatment of disorders induced by drugs or poisons is directed at the removal of the toxic substance from the body, management of agitation with minimal medication, adequate nutrition, monitoring of vital signs, uncovering of the reasons for the ingestion of substance, and supportive psychotherapy.

Health Education

A. Delirium

Teach patient and family that outcome is generally a full return to previous functioning level.

B. Dementia

1. Instruct and demonstrate ways to assist self in remembering, to avoid stress, and to maintain good health habits and activities of daily living.
2. Show family ways to offer emotional support to each other and ways to cope with stress of seeing older family member change.
3. Assist family in developing ways to combat disorientation (*e.g.,* appointment calendars, clocks, stable routines, set places for important items).
4. Assist family in identifying increasing anxiety in their loved one; signs are purposeless movements, verbalized desire to leave a situation, silence, decreasing ability to participate in interactions, and fidgeting. Offer ways to reduce anxiety.
5. Help family avoid anxiety-producing situations or limit amount of time person is in anxiety-producing situations.
6. Assist spouse in identifying problem areas, such as
   a. Loss of spouse as a marriage partner.
   b. Acceptance of the partner as he or she progressively deteriorates.

C. Disorders induced by specific causes

Instruct persons involved in ways to avoid cause or deal with consequence.

Commonly Associated Nursing Diagnoses

1. Aggression, inappropriate
2. Anxiety

3. Depressive behavior
4. Suspiciousness
5. Communication, impaired
6. Coping, ineffective individual, related to organic brain syndrome
7. Suicide, potential
8. Thought processes, alteration in
9. Self-care deficit: feeding, bathing/hygiene, dressing/grooming, toileting
10. Social isolation

Substance Use Disorders

Substance use disorders are a group of mental disorders manifested by impairments in social and occupational functions that are related to a regular use of specific substances that are intended to alter mood or behavior.

Definitions

A. Intoxication

A term used to indicate specific symptoms, including disturbed behavior associated with ingestion of substance.

B. Abuse

A term used to indicate a daily use of substance in order to function, intoxication, inability to stop use, and disturbed social and work behaviors (arrests, car accidents, absences from work, fights) for at least a 1-month period.

C. Dependence

A term used to indicate the presence of physiological dependence.

1. *Tolerance*—A term used to indicate that more of the substance is needed to obtain the same effect or that the same amount of the substance is not producing the same effect.
2. *Withdrawal*—A term used to indicate a syndrome following the absence of the usual intake of the substance. Symptoms of anxiety, insomnia, irritability, restlessness, and impaired attention along with symptoms related to the lack of the specific substance are present.

Incidence

1. Alcholism affects 7.5 to 10 million people and is considered by some to be the number one health problem.
   a. In other countries, 10% of people are reported to drink heavily.
   b. Problem drinking occurs most frequently in people under 25 years of age.
   c. Teenage drinking is an increasing problem.
      (1) Among teenagers, 3 million have drinking problems.
      (2) Approximately one third of high school seniors get drunk once weekly.
      (3) Car accidents related to alcohol are the number-one cause of death in this group.

    d. Women account for 30 to 50% of alcoholics but for only 20% of the population in treatment for this illness.

    e. Patients with alcohol-related conditions occupy 50% of hospital beds.

    f. Alcohol use decreases work productivity, increases health problems, and causes accidents.

2. Marijuana is the most frequent illicit drug used.

    a. It has been used by 27% of youth.

    b. Approximately 25% of 18- to 25-year-old people are at risk for the negative effects of its use.

3. Use of illicit drugs other than marijuana is found mostly among people who are 18 to 25 years old. Approximately 25% of the members of this group have tried cocaine and hallucinogens. Cocaine is the most popular drug of the 1980s.

4. Heroin addicts number 1 to 3 million.

5. Substance abuse is more common in men.

6. Barbiturate overdose is related to 6% of suicides.

7. Diazepam (Valium), alcohol, and heroin are the top three drugs used by patients seen in emergency departments.

Etiology

No known specific cause, but suggested hypotheses are

1. Genetic inheritance.

2. Environmental influences.

3. Psychodynamic theory—Emphasizes fixation at oral stage of development, such as failure to develop internal controls and continued insistence on immediate gratification.

4. Learning theory—The drugs produce an anesthesia and depressant/stimulant effect, and problems seem less pressing and real; behavior is then reinforced and continues.

5. Presence of a personality disorder.

6. Family-relationship problems.

7. Children who are having problems in school, having health problems, or being narcissistic.

8. Overdependence on mother and hostility towards father.

9. Peer pressure.

10. Familial association noted in alcoholism.

11. Physiological theories to explain dependence as the substance affecting the neurotransmitters or affecting cellular adaptation.

12. Overprescribed medication.

13. A drug pattern that may begin with alcohol and cigarette use, then progress to use of marijuana, followed by illicit drug use.

Clinical Manifestations of Selected Types Associated with Abuse and Dependence

A. Opiates, morphine, heroin

1. Taken orally, intravenously (needle tracts), and subcutaneously (skin pops and nodules).

2. Nonmedical use—To achieve pain relief and euphoria.
3. Intoxication—Pinpoint pupils, slow respirations, slow pulse, low blood pressure, hypothermia, drowsiness, euphoria, apathy, dysphoria, impairment in memory and attention.
4. Overdose
   a. Coma, shock, pinpoint pupils, respiratory depression.
   b. Treatment consists of administration of naloxone.
5. Withdrawal
   a. Symptoms occur within 1 week after last dose.
   b. Early signs—Restlessness, dilatation of pupils, sweating, tearing, runny nose, yawning, fever, and increase in pulse and respiration rates.
   c. Later signs—Muscle aches and spasms, GI symptoms, increased blood pressure, insomnia, anorexia, agitation.
6. Dependence
   a. Use of drug for an average of 9 years.
   b. A high death rate related to violent life-styles and physical complications.

B. Amphetamines
1. Taken orally, intravenously, or by inhalation.
2. Nonmedical use—To provide relief from fatigue, to assist with studying, to produce euphoria and sense of well-being, and to recover from hangover.
3. Intoxication
   a. Elation, talkativeness, pacing, hypervigilance, dilatation of pupils, tachycardia, increased blood pressure, GI symptoms, chills, perspiration, and sometimes persistent delusions or hallucinations.
   b. Similar to that experienced with cocaine.
4. Overdose—Convulsions, cardiovascular shock, hyperpyrexia.
5. Amphetamine delirium—Includes symptoms of delirium, changing affect, and frequent aggressive with violent behavior.
6. Withdrawal—Depression, anxiety, lethargy, disorientation, irritability, muscle spasms, GI symptoms sweating, headache.
7. Dependence
   a. Pattern is characteristically heavy use for several days or weeks (a "run"), followed by abstinence, which results in a "crash."
   b. This may continue for a year.

C. Barbiturates or similarly acting hypnotics (Valium, methaqualone)
1. Taken orally most frequently, but may be given IV.
2. Nonmedical use
   a. For treating nervousness, insomnia.
   b. For obtaining a high or sense of well-being.
3. Intoxication
   a. Slurred speech, unsteadiness, poor memory, and attention, impaired judgment, talkativeness, irritability, hostility, sexual aggressiveness.
   b. Similar to alcohol intoxication.

4. Overdose—Death is frequently by an accidental overdose or drug interaction.
5. Withdrawal—Anxiety, tremors, convulsions, postural hypotension, glabellar reflex (blinking continues despite tap on frontal bone between the eyebrows), psychotic state, nausea, vomiting, fever.
6. Dependence—Person may eventually cease taking the drug.

D. Cannabis (marihuana)

1. Can be smoked or ingested.
2. Nonmedical use—For obtaining a high and enhancing creativity.
3. Intoxication
   a. May be initial anxiety for 10 to 30 minutes, then euphoria, intensified perceptions, slowed time, apathy, tachycardia, dry mouth, increased appetite, passivity, drowsiness.
   b. Always conjunctival injection (bloodshot eyes due to dilation of arterioles).
   c. Lasts about 3 hours.
   d. Experience is affected by expectations of users.
4. Side effects include impairment of lung function, ovulation, sperm count and motility, driving skill, and immediate memory.
5. Death is rare.
6. Dependence
   a. Controversy surrounds this issue.
   b. Some people stop when impairment of functioning begins.

E. Alcohol

1. Taken orally in varying strengths in types of drinks.
2. Nonmedical use—To relax, to be life of the party and to have sense of being "sharp."
3. Intoxication—Slurred speech, unsteadiness, memory and attention problems, incoordination, talkativeness, irritability, depression, withdrawal, aggressive and sexual acts, nystagmus, flushed face, blackouts, blood level of alcohol 100 to 200 mg% and, potential for seizures. Blood alcohol level of 0.10% (100 mg%) constitutes intoxication according to law.
4. Overdose
   a. Unconsciousness with blood level of 400 mg/dl to 500 mg/dl
   b. Death with blood level of 600 mg/dl to 800 mg/dl with complications of respiratory depression.
5. Withdrawal
   a. Minor reactions occur 6 to 8 hours after no alcohol intake then increase within 24 to 36 hours. They include flushed face, sweating, bloodshot eyes, anorexia, nausea/vomiting, increased requests for sleeping medication or alcohol, tachycardia, and increased blood pressure.
   b. Seizures occur 7 to 48 hours after no alcohol intake.
   c. Alcohol withdrawal delirium (delirium tremens)
      (1) Usually occurs 72 to 96 hours after alcohol use is stopped.
      (2) Symptoms are coarse tremor of hands, feet, tongue, and eyelids;

slurred speech; vivid hallucinations; unpredictable or violent acts; confusion; disorientation; tachycardia; fever; high blood pressure; sweating; and dilated pupils.

(3) Mortality rate is 9% to 15%.

6. Long-term effects—Loss of self-respect, poor hygiene, alienation of friends and family, unemployment, child abuse, malnutrition, ulcers, heart problems, susceptibility to respiratory infections, hypertension, brain damage, cirrhosis of liver, Korsakoff's psychosis, and pancreatitis.

7. Dependence
   a. May continue throughout life.
   b. The sequence of developing dependence according to Jellineck's 1946 study of 2000 alcoholic men is as follows:[2]
      (1) Periodic excessive drinking
      (2) Blackouts
      (3) Sneaking drinks
      (4) Loss of control over drinking
      (5) Remorse and rationalization
      (6) Changing pattern of drinking as way to control consumption
      (7) Morning drinking
      (8) Binges lasting several days
      (9) Life centered on drinking and defeat that has been experienced

Clinical Manifestations of Selected Types Associated with Abuse

A. Cocaine

1. Taken by sniffing through nose, through injection, and through genitals.
2. Nonmedical use—To achieve "rush" of well-being and confidence, to be more talkative and energetic, and to assist in performance of sports and music.
3. Intoxication—Elation, talkativeness, pacing, hypervigilance, dilation of pupils, tachycardia, increased blood pressure and pulse, chills, perspiration, and transient delusions and hallucinations.
4. Death is rare.
5. Abuse
   a. Pattern may continue 2 to 8 months.
   b. Moral deterioration is frequently associated with its use.

B. Phencyclidine (PCP)

1. Taken orally, intravenously, or by sniffing or smoking.
2. Nonmedical use—To achieve some self-learning or social experience.
3. Intoxication
   a. Nystagmus (a very important finding), increased blood pressure and pulse, ataxia, dysarthria, diminished responsiveness to pain, euphoria, agitation, anxiety, grandiosity, emotional lability, synesthesias, slowing of time, unpleasantness, blank stare, hallucinations, paranoid ideation, violent acts (including self-mutilation), extreme unpredictability.
   b. May last 5 days.

    c. Recovery occurs in several days to 2 weeks because PCP is a long-acting drug that has a high concentration in the CNS. Patient slowly becomes less assaultive, suspicious, and agitated.

    d. After the PCP symptoms have resolved, the patient may begin to experience a major depression.

4. Death is possible but rare.

C. Hallucinogens (LSD, DMT, mescaline)

1. Taken orally or smoked.
2. Nonmedical use—To elevate mood.
3. Hallucinogen hallucinosis—Synesthesias, visual hallucinations, illusions, depersonalization, derealization, intensified perceptions, dilation of pupils, tachycardia, sweating, blurring of vision, tremors, incoordination.
4. "Bad trip": A panic state lasting 8 to 12 hours.
5. Flashbacks
    a. Are a repetition of an aspect of the drug-induced experience, such as a flash of light or seeing a figure lasting seconds or minutes occurring days to weeks after ingestion.
    b. Marihuana smoking is frequently associated with flashbacks.
6. Abuse: Generally occurs for brief periods only.

Treatment

A. Varied problems

1. There is no one treatment to deal with the varied problems with which a patient presents.
2. Treatment problems include inability to see need for help, attitude of public toward drug use, denial, poor motivation to continue treatment goals, issue of abstinence versus controlled drinking, and negative attitudes generated in staff.
3. Family issues that may need to be resolved are
    a. Need to contain negative feelings within self as way to maintain the family; problem is ignored.
    b. "Games" played by family members.
    c. Focus on a person as the problem.
    d. Lack of communication and poor use of problem-solving skills.

B. Complications

Treatment of associated complications, such as malnutrition, infections from use of contaminated needles and syringes, allergic reactions, erosion of nasal septum from cocaine "snorting" (placement of cocaine in nose), hepatitis, gastritis, neuropathy, venereal disease, cirrhosis, pancreatitis, family disruption, and social problems.

C. Detoxification programs

1. Alcohol user—Antianxiety drugs, particularly diazepam and chlordiazepoxide, are used to lessen symptoms of withdrawal. Antipsychotic drugs may be used to treat hallucinosis, but observation for seizures, orthostatic hypotension, or temperature regulation problems is then essential. Seizure

medication is usually not given prophylactically. The key to treatment of delirium tremens is prevention. In this withdrawal state, intensive medical care is indicated.

2. Opiate user
   a. Methadone is given in progressively decreasing doses for help with the withdrawal symptoms.
   b. Other therapies may be offered.
3. Barbiturate user—Decrease barbiturate dosages to levels at which only a mild withdrawal state will be produced. Procedure requires careful monitoring.
4. PCP user
   a. A patient in the acute intoxication state generally requires hospitalization because of the great danger to self and others.
   b. Treatment focuses on managing the environment to prevent overstimulation and to maintain safety of patient and others; on reducing psychosis with neuroleptics; on promoting excretion of PCP by giving cranberry juice or ammonium chloride tablets; on maintaining interpersonal contact to reassure patient; and on support of life functions with high-calorie and high-carbohydrate diet, multivitamins, fluids, and so on.

D. Therapeutic communities

1. Alcoholics Anonymous
   a. Group is organized to provide group support of abstinence based on a 12-step program and on the basic beliefs that "once an alcoholic, always an alcoholic" and that every alcoholic needs help to stop drinking.
   b. There is also an organization for spouses of alcoholics, Al-Anon.
2. Synanon, Phoenix House—Groups organized to assist the addict through a highly structured program and some degree of isolation from others.

E. Maintenance program for addicts

1. Purpose is to assist patient in achieving a comfortable state, but without feelings of euphoria experienced with opiate use.
2. Controversy exists over the 2-year limit on the maintenance program for the individual addict.

F. Use of deterrents

1. Disulfiram (Antabuse)
   a. Drug is taken daily and causes toxic reaction if alcohol is taken also.
   b. Symptoms include flushed feeling, weakness, nausea, low blood pressure.
2. Narcotic antagonists (naloxone, cyclazocine, naltrexone)—A group of drugs used to block the effects of opiates.

G. Anxiety and depression

Antianxiety and antidepressant medications are given to assist with the symptoms of anxiety and depression.

H. Psychotherapy

1. Psychotherapy in various forms is recommended for patients experiencing alcoholism to deal with problems of denial, reasons for drinking behaviors, and avoidance of sobriety.
2. Insight therapy has poor rate of success. Behavior therapy—which helps patient learn not to drink, learn alternatives to drinking, develop social skills, learn relaxation techniques, and so on—has a greater success rate. Crisis intervention approaches are useful.
3. Treatment of drug dependence focuses more frequently on achieving a drug-free state than on dealing with emotional problems that preceded drug use.

Health Education

1. Support primary prevention activities, such as
   a. Development of alternatives to drug use (*e.g.*, recreational activities).
   b. Public laws to deter drug use and availability.
   c. Recognition by society of the harmfulness of drug use. Note newspaper and magazine articles, TV programs, development of clubs to fight drug use, and so on.
   d. Education of the effects and consequences of long-term use.
2. Recognize particular importance of drug and alcohol education programs in school system that are designed to prevent abuse.
3. Teach signs and symptoms of intoxication, withdrawal, and/or dependence; associated physical problems that may develop; and available treatment resources. Assist in identifying changes needed in life-style. Assist family and/or friends in supporting patient; they may feel hopeless about treatment outcomes. Support groups exist for families of drug or alcohol patients.
4. Teach patient the numerous alcohol–drug interactions:
   a. Point out depressant effects of alcohol and barbiturates, minor and major tranquilizers, narcotics.
   b. Inform that sedative effects are enhanced by alcohol and antihistamines.
   c. Many other drugs have antagonistic, additive, or cross-tolerance interaction with alcohol; therefore, have patient carefully tell doctor all medications he is on, and encourage him to stop drinking.
5. Discuss with patient the increased risk for heart disease, tuberculosis, pneumonia, cirrhosis, neurological disorders, car accidents, committing murder, committing suicide, injury while falling, and exposure to extremes of temperature.
6. Help family use problem-solving approaches in dealing with crisis situations and in handling the possible long-term treatment process.

Commonly Associated Nursing Diagnoses

1. Anxiety
2. Depressive behavior
3. Self-care deficit: feeding, bathing/hygiene, dressing/grooming, toileting
4. Substance abuse (alcohol)

5. Substance abuse (drugs)
6. Coping, ineffective individual
7. Sensory/perceptual alteration: visual, auditory, kinesthetic, gustatory, tactile, olfactory
8. Suicide, potential
9. Family process, alteration in

Schizophrenic Disorders

Schizophrenia represents a group of mental disorders that present varied symptoms of disordered thinking and bizarre social behaviors.

Incidence

1. Schizophrenia affects approximately 1% of the total population (1 to 2 million); it is the most prevalent of the major psychoses.
2. The disorder affects adolescents and young adults.
3. There is an increased incidence in lower social class.
4. Patients with this diagnosis occupy 50% of hospital beds.
5. Prognosis: 25% recover completely, 50 to 65% have residual symptoms and relapses, and 10% remain ill.

Risk Factors

1. Family member with schizophrenia
2. Difficult delivery with trauma to brain of child
3. Children who are
   a. Highly individualistic in their thought processes.
   b. Overly dependent and obedient.
   c. Unable to enjoy life.
   d. Shy, withdrawn, and loners.
   e. Sensitive to separation.
   f. Unmanageable; prone to destructive, aggressive behavior.
   g. Truant from school.
4. Parents who are
   a. Hostile, very possessive, insensitive to needs of children
   b. Suspicious and inclined toward disturbances in thinking.
5. Illness
   a. Medical condition (*e.g.*, temporal lobe epilepsy)
   b. Drug abuse (*e.g.*, marihuana, PCP) and chemical factors (*e.g.*, MAO-B in blood platelets).
6. Abnormal eye pursuit movements

Etiology

No single cause, but hypotheses and research studies indicate several possible factors:
1. Hereditary factor
2. Genetic predisposition
3. Disturbance in neurotransmitter system
4. Intrauterine metabolic disorder

5. Slow virus
6. Premature birth with consequent immature body systems
7. Possible deviations of ego and superego development resulting in impairment of functioning; these deviations remain unproven hypotheses; deviations may be related to
   a. Increased sensitivity to stimuli or unpredictable regulatory system making it difficult for mothers to respond appropriately and for infant to feel safe and secure.
   b. Disturbed bond between mother and child and/or father and child.
   c. Developmental difficulties.
8. Disturbed family interaction patterns
   a. Borderline parents exhibit use of projection and splitting, making it problematic for the child to understand or adapt to his world.
   b. Marital schism and faulty familial communication. Child experiences double binds and maladaptive ways to deal with problems. What the child learns about interacting with others in the family cannot be transferred into the community, thus creating additional difficulties.
9. Environmental stresses, such as major crisis or migration

Clinical Manifestations

A. Early signs

1. Blocking or cutting off conversation; not responding as usual to friends, appearing aloof
2. Experiencing blackouts or other spells
3. Expressing various body symptom concerns
4. Forgetting and abandoning plans or life goals
5. Disregarding social customs and talking about abstract ideas such as love, creation, equality

B. Onset

An experience involving loss, separation, rejection; or use of LSD, marihuana, alcohol, amphetamine.

C. Acute phase

1. Hallucinations, especially auditory
   a. Voices are heard commenting in general.
   b. Voices may be saying, "You are this . . . You do that"; they may make obscene and threatening remarks or command the patient to do a violent act.
   c. Tactile and olfactory hallucinations may indicate temporal lobe epilepsy or presence of tumor. Cocaine abuse may cause tactile hallucinations.
   d. Visual hallucinations are seen in hysteria and schizophrenia, but they can also be indicators of organic disorders.

      ʔry disturbances, especially optical (*e.g.,* changing shapes and fig-

      of persecution, grandeur, or impending destruction

4. Autistic thinking characterized by being highly personal and not logical with perseveration, blocking, concretization, and loosening of associations
5. Speech characterized by incoherence, use of symbols, and concrete responses; possibly echolalia, flight of ideas, neologisms, inability or unwillingness to speak
6. Inappropriate behavior, such as grimacing, negativism, anergia (state of inaction), suggestibility, poor personal hygiene, few social manners
7. Blunting, ambivalence, and inappropriateness of affect

D. Residual phase

Symptoms of flat or blunted affect, rambling speech, poor hygiene and grooming, and distortion of some perceptual experiences may remain.

E. Relapse phase or stage of decompensation[3]
1. Feelings of being overwhelmed
2. Feelings of boredom, apathy
3. Disinhibition; impulsive expression of feelings
4. Psychotic disorganization with increasing perceptual and cognitive dysfunction, loss of identity, loss of self-control
5. Psychotic reaction with a decrease in anxiety and a psychotic organization of self

Selected Types

A. Catatonic schizophrenia

A disorder characterized by
1. Stuporous state in which person is mute, is negative, or complains in response to a request; is immobile; displays waxy flexibility; may retain urine and feces.
2. Excited state in which person is assaultive, aggressive, hyperactive, or agitated.

B. Disorganized schizophrenia

A disorder characterized by incoherence, foolishness, and regressive behavior.

C. Paranoid schizophrenia

A disorder characterized by delusions of persecution or grandeur.

D. Undifferentiated schizophrenia

A disorder characterized by a variety of symptoms found in several types.

Treatment

1. Relationship with therapist is vital. Therapist must be able to understand the patient, to offer him support and guidance, and to engage him in a therapeutic relationship and other treatment modalities.
2. Importance of social relationships in support of the patient during recovery

is being recognized. Self-concept is enhanced; approval is given even after the illness is experienced; opportunities for ventilation by patient and feedback from friends are present; and material help is given.

3. Family support and involvement are necessary. Expression of hostility, overinvolvement, and/or frequent criticism contribute to the recurrence of symptoms in the patient.
4. Treatment choices are related to the stage of the disease, the amount of regression, the availability of reality testing, the motivation for treatment, stress management skills, available resources, and the ability to relate to a therapist.
5. Long-term treatment of the patient involves programs that assist in many areas: basic needs for food, place to live, and clothing; assistance with medical problems; development of social and vocational skills; medication needs; and development of social support system. This requires collaboration among health professionals. Frequently, services are not readily available and patients seek help among themselves. A "ghettoization" of the chronically mental ill occurs.
6. A variety of therapies are available and are used to meet treatment goals designed for the individual patient.
   a. *Short hospitalization*—To assist with problems of dangerousness to self or others, of deviant behaviors that are increasingly abrasive to family and community, and of monitoring effects of drugs or other therapies.
   b. *Day treatment and outpatient treatment*—To provide help with problems arising from familial, work, and social situations while patient remains in the situations.
   c. *Outpatient treatment*—To provide aftercare, maintenance therapy, social support programs, and medication clinics.
   d. *Rehabilitation services*—To provide range of opportunities to increase skills in living, such as vocational rehabilitation, foster home care, halfway houses.
   e. *Milieu therapy*—To assist in counteracting the patient with chronic schizophrenica from withdrawing from society and dependence on an institutional life-style.
   f. *Drug therapy with antipsychotics*—To assist in ameliorating symptoms and in increasing patient's availability for psychotherapy.
   g. *Psychotherapy*—To assist patient in daily problems by exploration of relationships, sources of anxiety, and coping techniques.
   h. *Group therapy*—To offer support with problems encountered in everyday life.
   i. *Behavior therapy*—To assist with bizarre and disruptive behaviors in a variety of forms, such as token economy, and to provide social skills training.
   j. *Electroconvulsive therapy*—For patients with severe psychoses.
   k. *Psychoanalysis*—Is considered generally inappropriate because of intense relationship problems encountered and because of the relatively poor recovery rate.
   l. *Family therapy*—To assist in defining the problem as one concerning the entire family rather than one concerning the patient alone, to improve

communication, to clarify roles within family, to manage stress, and to assist in problem-solving.

Health Education

1. Teach patient and family the various ways to obtain help in improving work, educational, and social skills.
2. Explain that the potential for rehospitalization is approximately 20% to 50%; therefore, information and support are needed to continue aftercare plans and to decrease discouragement if rehospitalization becomes a reality.
3. Teach patient and family knowledge and skills involved in self-administration of medication; help patient tolerate and/or adapt to the side effects of the drugs.
4. Encourage patient and family to identify stress early and then to use problem-solving skills.
5. Advise family on how to supervise the patient's medication and how to respond to disturbing behaviors.
6. Provide information about the nature of schizophrenia and the treatments available.
7. Review and/or teach the basic health habits.
8. Stress the importance of not using illicit drugs and alcohol.

Commonly Associated Nursing Diagnoses

1. Manipulation
2. Noncompliance
3. Aggression, inappropriate
4. Communication, impaired
5. Anxiety
6. Suspiciousness
7. Impulsiveness
8. Sensory/perceptual alteration: visual, auditory, kinesthetic, gustatory, tactile, olfactory
9. Self-care deficit: feeding, bathing/hygiene, dressing/grooming, toileting
10. Coping, ineffective individual
11. Suicide, potential
12. Thought processes, alteration in
13. Self-concept, disturbance in: self-esteem, role performance, personal identity

Paranoid Disorders

Paranoid disorders represent a group of mental disorders manifested by delusions of jealousy and of persecution that are not explained by other psychiatric disorders.

Etiology

No known specific cause, but hypotheses and research suggest several factors:

1. Psychodynamic theory—Postulates the use of denial and projection as defenses against homosexual wishes as basis for delusions.

2. Childhood developmental deficits of failure to develop basic trust—Related to physical abuse, broken homes, and unpredictable parents or other forms of rejection.
3. Parental expectations of perfection and high achievement.
4. Stress situations involving lowering of self-esteem, increasing distrust, envy, isolation, and other factors leading to a delusional system that is a frightening but partially comforting

Clinical Manifestations of Selected Type
Paranoia
1. This disorder has a clear, logical, lasting delusional system.
2. Interpersonal relationships are poor because there is a basic mistrust of all.

Treatment
1. *Hospitalization*—Generally not indicated because person seldom seeks treatment, and community develops a tolerance for the odd behaviors. If delusions are causing person to behave in ways dangerous to self or others, hospitalization is indicated.
2. *Drug therapy* with antipsychotics.
3. *Psychotherapy*—Initially deals with the problem of establishing a trusting relationship and with immediate, concrete problems; later discussion involves delusions and the mistrust of others.

Commonly Associated Nursing Diagnoses
1. Suspiciousness
2. Aggression, inappropriate
3. Thought processes, alteration in

Affective Disorders
Affective disorders are a group of mental disorders that present mainly with symptoms of mood disturbance with associated changes in thinking and behavior.

Incidence
1. Most common disorder grouping in adults; bipolar disorder in about 600,000 cases per year and unipolar depressive disorder in 1.5 million cases per year.
2. Females outnumber males 2 to 1.
3. Estimated 20% to 50% of people over 65 years of age experience depression.
4. There are only 20% to 25% of people with depression seeking treatment.
5. Bipolar disorder occurs before age 30 years; depression occurs at any age.
6. An underdiagnosis of bipolar disorder in United States may exist.
7. Depression occurring for the first time after the age of 40 years frequently indicates underlying physical illness.
8. Depression is frequently associated with other medical disorders or treatment:

a. Side effects of some drugs (*e.g.,* drugs used in the treatment of high blood pressure)
b. Endocrine diseases (hypothyroidism, Addison's disease)
c. Neurological diseases (brain tumors, Parkinson's disease)
d. Cancer
e. Alcoholism

Etiology

No known one specific cause, but hypotheses and research indicate several factors:
1. Genetic factors
2. Disturbance in neurotransmitter system involving norepinephrine, serotonin, dopamine, acetylcholine.
3. Disturbance of steroid hormones
4. Stressful life events prior to onset of illness
5. Lack of social support (an important variable)
6. Psychodynamic view of depression and mania with hostility, turned against self or projected to others, being the primary factor; early experiences of separation and loss of parents
7. Ego adaptive view of depression as ego state response to separation and loss
   a. Avoidance of overt anger to prevent endangerment of relationships in which dependency needs are met
   b. Idealization of another with consequence that there is no need for anger
   c. Implication of anger involving autonomy, which the depressed person does not understand
8. Cognitive view of depression with individual viewing himself, the future, and the current experience in a negative way
9. Family interaction patterns in which child experiences high expectations of achievement by parents and little approval for being self

Clinical Manifestation of Selected Types

A. Major depression
1. Symptoms include sadness, apathy, feelings of worthlessness, self-blame, thoughts of suicide, desire to escape, avoidance of simple problems, anorexia, weight loss, lessened interest in sex, sleeplessness, reduction in activity, or ceaseless activity.
2. In infants and older children, symptoms are refusal to eat, listlessness, lack of activity, fear of the death of a parent, fear of separation from parents.
3. In adolescents, symptoms are social isolation, negative attitude, sulkiness, feelings of being unappreciated, acting out in antisocial ways.

B. Bipolar disorder
   A disorder in which there are alternating periods of depression and mania.
1. *Bipolar disorder, manic episode*—Symptoms include hyperactivity, speech pressure, grandiosity, manipulativeness, irritability, euphoria, mood liability, hypersexuality, delusions, assaultiveness, and sleeplessness.

2. *Bipolar disorder, depressive episode*—Symptoms are the same as those of major depression.

C. Dysthymic disorder

A new diagnostic category for disorders in which person experiences for at least 2 years a depressed mood, no pleasure in activities of daily living, an impairment in social skills, and numerous bodily complaints.

Treatment

1. *Hospitalization*—Used in acute mania and in depression when there is evidence of poor judgment, weight loss, insomnia, and lack of emotional support.
2. *Electroconvulsive therapy*—Used in severe depression or mania.
3. *Drug therapy* with antidepressants or antimanic drugs—Neuroleptics may be used to assist in controlling the violent behavior seen in manic state.
4. *Psychotherapy*—Used in various forms to deal with issues of dependency and manipulation, of need to detoxify, of loss experience, and of self-destructiveness.
5. *Cognitive psychotherapy*—Focuses on the correction of negative errors in thinking. Efficacy of cognitive therapy is equal to that of drug therapy.
6. *Behavioral therapy*—Focuses on developing ways to reward behavior and on learning to experience pleasure; assertiveness training; and social skills training (*e.g.,* how to participate in social conversation).
7. *Maintenance of social supports*—Focuses on encouraging family support of patient and on facilitating communication with the patient.
8. *Prevention of suicide*
9. *Vigorous exercise*—Associated with improvement in patients who are moderately depressed.

Health Education

1. Help family cope with their feelings of fear, frustration, anger, and guilt toward the patient.
2. Provide information about affective disorders, major treatments, and prognosis.
3. Assist family and patient in learning about antidepressants or lithium being prescribed; help them adapt to side effects of the medication.
4. Discuss signs of increasing depression and danger of suicide.
5. Assist patient in seeking information from self and others to identify the prodromal stage of manic state.
6. Assist patient and family in learning ways to manage stress.

Commonly Associated Nursing Diagnoses

1. Aggression, inappropriate
2. Manipulation
3. Manic behavior
4. Depressive behavior
5. Noncompliance
6. Suicide, potential

7. Coping, ineffective individual, related to maturational crisis
8. Coping, ineffective individual, related to situational crisis
9. Thought processes, alteration in
10. Self-care deficit: feeding, bathing/hygiene, dressing/grooming, toileting

Anxiety Disorders

Anxiety disorders are a group of mental disorders in which anxiety is the main concern.

Incidence

1. Panic disorder and generalized anxiety disorder may affect 5% of the population.
2. Obsessive-compulsive disorder may affect 0.05% of the population.
3. Phobic disorder may affect 8% of the population; following are some common phobias:
   a. *Agoraphobia*—Fear of open places; this is the most common phobia.
   b. *Acrophobia*—Fear of heights.
   c. *Claustrophobia*—Fear of enclosed places.
   d. *Animal phobias*
   e. *Social phobia*

Etiology

1. Psychodynamic theory views anxiety as arising from conflicts that are usually sexual and aggressive.
   a. Types
      (1) Superego anxiety (*e.g.,* fear of being found guilty)
      (2) Castration anxiety (*e.g.,* fear of bodily mutilation or decrease of abilities and skills)
      (3) Separation anxiety (*e.g.,* fear of loss of significant relationship)
      (4) Impulse anxiety (*e.g.,* fear of loss of control of impulses)
   b. Obsessive-compulsive disorder arises during anal developmental stage; mental mechanisms used are undoing, isolation, and reaction formation
   c. Phobic disorder is characterized by use of mechanisms of displacement and avoidance to deal with castration anxiety and oedipal drives.
2. Behavioral theory views the anxiety disorders as automatic learned responses to situations that are anxiety-provoking.
3. Other theories stress the importance of separation anxiety and aggressive impulses.

Clinical Manifestations of Selected Types

A. Panic disorder

Characterized by acute anxiety episode of intense terror and dread and by awareness of palpitation and tachycardia, chest pain, and air hunger.

B. Generalized anxiety disorder

Characterized by chronic anxiety (6 months) with restlessness, irritability, dry mouth, sweating of palms, GI symptoms, insomnia, and problems in concentration.

C. Obsessive-compulsive disorder

1. Characterized by a persistent idea or impulse that is neither acceptable nor controllable, anxious feelings, and attempts to resist the impulse.
2. Compulsive acts may be one act or complex rituals.

D. Phobic disorder

Characterized by an intense fear of an object (simple phobia), of a situation (agoraphobia), or of functioning in situations (social phobia).

Treatment

1. *Psychotherapy*—Used in various forms, with focus on analyzing unconscious conflicts, on interpersonal conflicts, or on only a supportive measure.
2. *Behavioral therapy*—Used with systematic desensitization, flooding, and reinforced practice to deal with anxiety-provoking stimuli. Has empirical support for its effectiveness.
3. *Cognitive therapy*—Helps patient's cognitive process relabel anxiety-producing aspects of the phobic situation and change negative statements about self.
4. *Drug therapy*—Antidepressant drugs are used.
5. *Relaxation techniques*
6. *Hospitalization*—Used for short periods if symptoms become intense and family's ability to offer support at that time is limited.
7. Focus on phobia as main treatment concern may lead to lack of awareness of frequently associated problems, such as depression, chronic anxiety, sexual problems, social isolation, presence of several phobias, work problems.

Health Education

1. Instruct patient with phobic disorder or obsessive-compulsive disorder that the condition may tend to be chronic.
2. Teach patient and family ways to deal with incapacities and inconveniences created by the disorders.
3. Teach patient relaxation techniques.
4. Teach patient ways to monitor self for increasing anxiety.

Commonly Associated Nursing Diagnoses

1. Anxiety
2. Ritualistic behavior
3. Depressive behavior
4. Guilt
5. Physical symptoms, inappropriate use of
6. Coping, ineffective individual
7. Coping, ineffective individual, related to situational crisis
8. Social isolation

Somatoform Disorders

Somatoform disorders are a group of mental disorders characterized by multiple somatic complaints with no physical illness.

Etiology

1. Etiology in somatization disorders is unknown.
2. Etiology in conversion disorders involves
    a. Fixation of development at Oedipus complex with resulting sexual conflicts and symptoms.
    b. Self-preservation drives to be protected and to escape.
    c. Pathological reactions and responses to environmental stress.

Clinical Manifestations of Selected Types

A. Somatization disorder

Characterized by symptoms of fatigue, nausea and vomiting, bowel problems, headaches, and fainting and by the dramatics and emotionality involved in describing problems.

B. Conversion disorder

Characterized by abnormal movements or paralysis of parts with no relation to specific nerve involvement, anesthesias, and symptoms of physical illness. Early signs of a neurological disorder may be called a conversion disorder.

Treatment

1. *Psychoanalysis*—Focuses on dynamics of repression.
2. *Psychotherapy*—Focuses on symptom alleviation and supportive techniques.
3. *Drug therapy*—Antianxiety drugs are used.

Health Education

1. Teach patient that symptoms may recur in stressful situations.
2. Help patient focus on returning to independence, and support family in allowing freedom of activities.
3. Instruct patient and families that having numerous types of treatments focused on the physical illness is not useful.

Commonly Associated Nursing Diagnoses

1. Anxiety
2. Physical symptoms, inappropriate use of
3. Noncompliance
4. Coping, ineffective individual, related to situational crisis
5. Coping, ineffective individual, related to maturational crisis
6. Substance abuse (alcohol)
7. Substance abuse (drugs)

Dissociative Disorders

Dissociative disorders are a group of mental disorders presenting as a temporary alteration in conscious awareness, identity, personality, and behavior.

Etiology

Psychodynamic theory states that dissociation is the mental mechanism used to deal with severe anxiety; also, conflicts arising from Oedipal and pre-Oedipal stages affect ego development.

Clinical Manifestations of Selected Type

Psychogenic amnesia
1. This is the most common form and is characterized by abrupt inability to recall pertinent information.
2. It frequently is associated with physical injury.

Treatment

Brief, immediate psychotherapy with emphasis on assisting recall to prevent material from becoming inaccessible to recall.

Health Education

Assist patient in seeking the brief psychiatric help needed.

Commonly Associated Nursing Diagnoses

1. Anxiety
2. Coping, ineffective individual

Personality Disorders

Personality disorders are a group of mental disorders characterized by life-long patterns of maladaptive responses to stress, by problems in developing work behaviors and intimate relationship behaviors, and by the capacity to perpetuate interpersonal problems and to annoy others.

Incidence

About 5% to 15% of the adult population with higher percentages in areas where socially impaired live.

Etiology

1. Not much is known about the causes.
2. A genetic factor is possible.
3. Disturbance in early childhood involving presence of inconsistent, neglectful parents is common.

Clinical Manifestations

1. Commonly used defense mechanisms are fantasy, isolation, dissociation, projection, somatization, splitting, and passive-aggressive behavior.
2. Person perceives self as extremely important and powerful.
3. Formation of dependent and demanding relationships.
4. Creation of entangled interpersonal relationships.

Selected Types

A. Paranoid personality disorder

Characterized by a history of mistrust of others.

B. Schizoid personality disorder

Characterized by history of withdrawal from society.

C. Histrionic personality disorder

Characterized by history of dramatic displays of emotions that include temper tantrums and suicide threats, of attention-seeking behaviors, of a desire for activity, and of brief relationships with others.

D. Antisocial personality disorder

Characterized by history of antisocial behavior involving courts, prisons, and health and welfare agencies.

E. Borderline personality disorder

1. Characterized by history of instability of affect; of impulsivity; of periods of intense anger; of intense, clinging relationships; and of unpredictable self-destructive acts.
2. Involves use of primitive defenses: splitting (people and world are viewed as good or bad), projective identification, and denial.
3. Occurs rarely, accounting for 1 to 5% of outpatient cases. Patient is remembered because of management problems he presents and the intense feelings aroused by him in staff.
4. Etiology is unknown, but hereditary factors exist and intense separation anxiety is perhaps related to parental neglect or exclusion.

F. Compulsive personality disorder

Characterized by history of orderliness, obstinateness, parsimony, emotional constriction, rigidity, indecisiveness, devotion to a task, and overconcern with rules and morals.

G. Passive-aggressive personality disorder

Characterized by history of resistance to most expectations involved in social and work settings and by procrastination, forgetfulness, and inefficiency.

Treatment

1. Treatment is very difficult because of the anxiety generated with responses of anger, defensiveness, and authoritarianism in therapist and staff. In addition, patient does not perceive self as sick.
2. Psychotherapy is helpful and can be
   a. *Long-term* treatment with focus on personality change.
   b. *Short-term* treatment with focus on adaptation; involves support and guidance with problems of living, assistance with limiting contact with situations that provoke problems, and help with developing personal assets.
3. Self-help groups are useful because person requires more support than any one person can provide.
4. Drug therapy involves use of antianxiety agents, of antipsychotics during psychotic episodes, and of antidepressants; there is no one specific medication.

Health Education

Instruct patient to become aware of the consequences of his behavior, and support his attempts to be involved in psychotherapy.

Commonly Associated Nursing Diagnoses

1. Manipulation
2. Impulsive behavior
3. Aggression, inappropriate
4. Noncompliance
5. Suspiciousness
6. Substance abuse (alcohol)
7. Substance abuse (drugs)
8. Coping, ineffective individual

SELECTED TREATMENT MODALITIES

Hospitalization

1. This is the treatment of choice when patient is acting suicidal, homicidal, or psychotic. A variety of treatment approaches can be used to assist the patient (*e.g.,* medication regimens; individual, group, and family therapies; and occupational and recreational therapies).
2. Most patients are treated on a voluntary basis because they are seeking treatment like any medical patient. However, some are admitted for emergency observation. After a time specified by state law (3 to 30 days), the patient can be committed for a stated period of time or indefinitely.
3. Short-term hospitalization (about 30 days) is a proven effective treatment for schizophrenia as opposed to long-term, intensive, analytically oriented hospitalization.
4. Crisis centers, day treatment centers, out-patient clinics, and home visits by nurses are other alternatives to hospitalization.
5. Feelings of nervousness, depression, restlessness, anxiety, and general dissatisfaction are reported as prodromal signs of relapse by friends and relatives of patients.
6. Several attempts to be admitted to a hospital and emotional distress and concerns are associated with rehospitalization more frequently than violent and psychotic behavior are.

Psychotherapy

A. Psychoanalysis (Freud)

1. Use of unconscious material, dream analysis, free association, interpretation, and transference to assist patient in achieving reorganization of his personality.
2. May extend over a period of 1 to 7 years.

B. Psychotherapy (Sullivan)

1. Use of relationship with analyst to focus on interpersonal relationship and communication process.
2. Dream analysis, free association, interpretation, and transference also are used to assist the individual.

C. Psychotherapy (Rogers)

Use of empathetic understanding, concreteness, self-exploration, and positive regard to encourage individual towards self-actualization.

D. Cognitive therapy (Beck)

1. Use of guided discovery to assist patient in focusing on dysfunctional thoughts or behaviors and analyzing them and in performing tasks.
2. Strategy for behavior change is based on interrupting the sequence of cognition, imagery, and affect.
3. Method has been studied and proven useful in depression.

E. Rational-emotive psychotherapy, RET (Ellis)

1. Therapist teaches person to use an "ABCDE" method for achieving his goals.
2. *A* is for activating experience by actively fantasizing experience to determine emotional consequence.
3. *B* is for belief system that a person notes as he allows self to feel uncomfortable.
4. *C* is for confronting irrational beliefs by using positive imagery.
5. *D* is for disputing irrational beliefs.
6. *E* is for effecting a change in beliefs and behavior.

F. Interpersonal therapy, IPT (Klerman)

Focus is on interpersonal transactions that have not gone well and on the development of specific strategies for coping with internal and external stress.

G. Transactional analysis (Berne)

1. Use of concepts of parent, child, and adult to describe ego states; use of transaction and games to view interactions with others.
2. Goal is to obtain the adult ego state of "I'm OK—You're OK" or a game-free relationship.

H. Reality therapy (Glaser)

Focus is on acceptance of reality and responsibility for self with the therapist who is involved in loving and teaching.

I. Supportive psychotherapy

Use of techniques to achieve other ways for control of impulses, to strengthen defenses, or to maintain adaptation.

J. Crisis therapy

1. Focus is on offering emotional support, providing for catharsis, communicating hope, setting model for action, listening selectively for material for assessment, providing factual information, setting limits on acting-out behavior, writing out contract, and formulating problem in terms of precipitating factors, background problems, and available coping mechanism.
2. Duration is one to six sessions.

K. Brief psychotherapy

1. Consists of one to 20 sessions involving techniques to help patient relate present situation to past experiences in order to assist him in removal of specific symptoms.
2. Outcome is related to experience of trust in the therapist relationship.

Group Psychotherapy

Selected persons are placed in a group of 4 to 10 people guided by a trained therapist to effect personality change or to assist with problems affecting mental health.

1. *Analytic group*—Leader uses psychoanalytic concepts to produce change.
2. *Sullivanian group*—Leader uses interpersonal theory to explore problems and eliminate maladaptations.
3. *Bion group*—Leader uses concepts concerning group life, including basic assumptions, to interpret group phenomena.
4. *Transactional group*—Leader focuses on games and not on determining causes of problems or on uncovering unconscious material to achieve "cure."
5. *Gestalt group (Perls)*—Leader uses rules and games to assist person in acknowledging immediate feelings and to prevent their avoidance in order to restore the person to a sense of wholeness.
6. *Psychodrama (Moreno)*
   a. This is a method offering opportunity for problem-solving through enactment of conflict situation.
   b. It involves a protagonist who acts out the situation, a director who assists in the exploration of the situation, an auxiliary who acts as a person in the protagonist's life, and an audience.
   c. Many techniques are used to promote involvement and analysis; some are soliloquy, self-presentation, mirror, role reversal, and double.
7. *Bibliotherapy*—Involves use of literature, films, and person's own creative writing with group discussion to promote self-knowledge and integration of thoughts and feelings.
8. *Self-help groups*—Focus on prevention of additional problems and further treatment by sharing and receiving help with problem-solving and coping skills from other members. About 500 groups exist.

Family Therapy

1. *Structural model (Minuchin)*
   a. Therapist seeks to alter the family structure because changes in the family structure will alter behavior and the psychic processes.
   b. Therapist uses joining operations as he recreates communication patterns.
2. *Bowen therapy*—Therapist assists family members in achieving differentiation and in reducing reactivity.

Electroconvulsive Therapy (ECT)

ECT is a series of 8 to 12 treatments, given with the patient under anesthesia and muscle relaxants, involving application of electrical current to the brain in order to produce convulsions; a monthly maintenance treatment is administered in some cases. It is indicated in severe cases of depression, psychoses, catatonia, and mania.

1. Studies have demonstrated its safety (mortality rate of 1/25,000) and effectiveness in the treatment of depression and have shown that results with this method are comparable to those obtained with antidepressant medications. Two important characteristics are its rapid action and its effectiveness after drug treatment has failed.
2. Behavioral changes are probably the result of biochemical changes in brain function.
3. Contraindication is presence of brain tumor.
4. Treatment preparation involves physical examination; lab tests; spine radiographs, if indicated; full, informed consent of patient; nothing by mouth after midnight; voiding prior to treatment; and removal of dentures.
5. Fractures or dislocations and pulmonary aspiration are the most frequent complications.
6. Patients need an adequate explanation of the treatment procedure so that fears are allayed and misinformation prevalent in society is corrected; preparation for memory loss should be made.
7. Patient will have amnesia for the treatment procedure and will experience some transient memory loss.
8. Immediately afterwards, the patient may be confused, drowsy, and euphoric or flat in affect. Some patients experience headaches, muscle pains, and nausea.
9. Orientation to time and space should be provided.
10. Communicating the expectation that the patient may assume daily activities may help promote more normal levels of activity in the patient.
11. Memory impairment for events prior to treatment and during treatment period may remain in some patients.

Activity Therapy

1. *Occupational therapy*—Use of selected activities (painting, pottery, leather work, crocheting, hammering, shopping, washing clothes, budgeting, etc.) to improve general performance, to learn essential skills of living, and to assist in symptom reduction.
2. *Recreation therapy*
   a. Use of recreational activities (social, sports, games, hobbies, arts, crafts, service activities, outdoor sports, etc.) in treatment of behavior.
   b. Special emphasis on resocialization, reality orientation, and involvements when working with psychiatric patients.
3. *Dance therapy*—Use of rhythmic movements and interaction to express emotions, thereby increasing awareness of body and ego strength.

Other Modalities

A. Sex therapy (Masters and Johnson)

Use of desensitizing techniques to increase sexual pleasure and arousal and to demystify sex.

B. Assertiveness training

Teaching of skills to assist people in getting what they want in a firm, effective, and useful manner as opposed to an aggressive manner, in which emotions are expressed in destructive, aggressive ways.

C. Biofeedback

Feedback of functioning of autonomic system through instruments that pick up electrical potentials; assists patient in gaining control of heart rate, blood pressure, skin temperature, and muscle tension.

D. Milieu therapy

Use of open door, homelike furnishings, high staff–patient ratio, patient government, democratic decision-making, ward–staff initiative, high interaction level with patients, and shared responsibility among patients to improve patient behavior.

E. Token economy

Use of positive reinforcement in form of tokens and extinction of undesirable behaviors by ignoring or being fined tokens to achieve behavior change.

F. Hypnosis

Use of techniques such as repetitive suggestion to induce state of altered consciousness or intense concentration to provide additional data for diagnosis and treatment; it in itself does not constitute treatment.

G. Relaxation techniques

Use of breathing, muscle, and autogenic exercises to relax and thereby reduce anxiety. Examples are listening to music, allowing thought to move freely, systematically contracting and relaxing body parts, closing the eyes, concentrating on some imaginary object just outside self, and breathing slowly several times.

REFERENCES

1. American Psychiatric Association: Diagnostic and Statistical Manual of Mental Disorders, 3rd ed. Washington DC, American Psychiatric Association, 1980
2. Jellinek EM: Phases in the drinking history of alcoholics. New Haven, CT, Hillhouse Press, 1946
3. Docherry JP et al: Stages of onset of schizophrenic psychosis. Am J Psychiatry 135, No. 4: 420–426, 1978

Bibliography

CONCEPTS OF MENTAL HEALTH AND MENTAL ILLNESS

Books

Aguilera DC, Messick JM: Crisis Intervention: Theory and Methodology, 4th ed. St Louis, CV Mosby, 1982

American Psychiatric Association: Diagnostic and Statistical Manual of Mental Disorders, 3rd ed. Washington DC, American Psychiatric Association, 1980

Atkinson RL, Atkinson RC, Hilgard ER: Introduction to Psychology, 8th ed. New York, Harcourt, Brace, Jovanovich, 1983

Bachrach LL: The homeless mentally ill and mental health services: An analytical review of the literature. In Lamb HR (ed): The Homeless Mentally Ill, A Task Force Report of the American Psychiatric Association. Washington DC, American Psychiatric Association, 1984

Bandura A. Principles of Behavior Modification. New York, Holt, Rinehart & Winston, 1969

Barchas JD, Berger PA, Ciaranello RD, Elliott GR: Psycho-Pharmacology: From Theory to Practice. New York, Oxford University Press, 1977

Beck A: Cognitive Therapy and Emotional Disorders. New York, International Universities Press, 1976

Bloom BL: Community Mental Health: A General Introduction, 2nd ed. Monterey, CA, Brooks Cole, 1984

Bootzin RR, Acocella JR: Abnormal Psychology: Current Perspectives. New York, Random House, 1984

Bowen M: Family Therapy in Clinical Practice. New York, Jason Aronson, 1978

Brenner C: An Elementary Textbook of Psychoanalysis, rev. ed. New York, Anchor Press, 1974

Clausen JA, Pfeffer NG, Huffine CL: Help-Seeking Behavior in Severe Mental Illness. In Mechanic D (ed): Symptoms, Illness, Behavior, and Help-Seeking. New Brunswick, NJ, Rutgers University Press, 1982

Erikson E: Childhood and Society. New York, WW Norton, 1964

Erikson E: Identity: Youth and Crisis. New York, WW Norton, 1968

Erikson E: Insight and Responsibility. New York, WW Norton, 1968

Erikson E: Toys and Reasons: Stages in the Ritualization of Experience. New York, WW Norton, 1977

Erikson E: Identity and the Life Cycle. New York, WW Norton, 1979

Ford DH, Urban HB: Systems of Psychotherapy. New York, John Wiley & Sons, 1963

Frankl VE: Man's Search for Meaning: An Introduction to Logotherapy. Boston, Beacon Press, 1963

Green RK, Schaefer AB: Forensic Psychology: A Primer for Legal and Mental Health Professionals. Springfield, IL, Charles C Thomas, 1984

Gurman AS, Kniskern DP (eds): Handbook of Family Therapy. New York, Brunner-Mazel, 1981

Hagerty BK: Psychiatric-Mental Health Assessment. St Louis, CV Mosby, 1984

Haley J: Problem Solving Therapy. San Francisco, Jossey-Bass, 1977

Haley J: Leaving Home. New York, McGraw-Hill, 1980

Jahoda M: Current Concepts of Positive Mental Health. New York, Basic Books, 1958

Johnson HC: The biological basis of psychopathology. In Turner FJ (ed): Adult Psychopathology: A Social Work Perspective. New York, Free Press, 1984

Kaslow FW (ed): The International Book of Family Therapy. New York, Brunner-Mazel, 1982

Koldjeski D: Community Mental Health Nursing. New York, John Wiley & Sons, 1984

Laird J, Allen J: Family theory and practice. In Rosenblatt A, Waldfogel D (eds): Handbook of Clinical Social Work. San Francisco, Jossey-Bass, 1983

Lamb HR (ed): The Homeless Mentally Ill, A Task Force Report of the American Psychiatric Association. Washington DC, American Psychiatric Association, 1984

Maslow AH (ed): Motivation of Personality, 2nd ed. New York, Harper & Row, 1970

Minuchin S: Families and Family Theory. Cambridge, MA, Harvard University Press, 1974

Mundt LB: Mental health treatment methods. In Austin MJ, Hershey WE (eds): Handbook on Mental Health Administration. San Francisco, Jossey-Bass, 1982

National Institute of Mental Health: Mental Health, United States, 1983. Taube CA, Barrett SA (eds): DHHS Pub No (ADM)83-1275. Rockville, MD, The Institute, 1983

Nicholi A (ed): The Harvard Guide to Modern Psychiatry. Cambridge, MA, Belknap Press, 1978

Pincus JH, Tucker GJ: Behavioral Neurology, 2nd ed. New York, Oxford University Press, 1978

Rogers C: A theory of therapy, personality and interpersonal relationships as developed in the client-centered framework. In Koch S (ed): Psychology, A Study of Science. New York, McGraw-Hill, 1963

Satir V: Conjoint Family Therapy, rev. ed. Palo Alto, CA, Science and Behavior Books, 1967

Shapiro SA: Contemporary Theories of Schizophrenia: Review and Synthesis. New York, McGraw-Hill, 1981

Snyder SH: Biological Aspects of Mental Disorder. New York, Oxford University Press, 1980

Subcommittee of the Joint Commission on Public Affairs. Werner A (chmn) et al: A Psychiatric Glossary, 5th ed. Washington, DC, Am Psychiatric Assoc, 1984

Sullivan HS: The Interpersonal Theory of Psychiatry. New York, WW Norton, 1953

Vaillant GE: Adaptation to Life. Boston, Little, Brown, 1977

Watzlawick P, Beavin J, Jackson D: Pragmatics of Human Communication. New York, WW Norton, 1967

Watzalwick P, Weakland CE, Fisch R: Change: Principles of Problem Formation and Problem Resolutions. New York, WW Norton, 1974

Wlliams A, Johnson J: Mental Health in the 21st Century. Lexington, Lexington Books, 1979

Wolpe J: The Practice of Behavior Therapy. Oxford, Pergamon Press, 1969

Articles

Caplan G: An approach to preventive intervention in child psychiatry. Can J Psychiatry. 25(8):671–682, 1980

Caplan G: Mastery of stress: psychosocial aspects. Am J Psychiatry 138(4):413–420, 1981

Clarkin JF, Glick ID: Recent developments in family therapy: a review. Hosp Community Psychiatry 33(7):550–556, 1982

Greenley JR: Social factors, mental illness and psychiatric care: recent advances from a sociological perspective. Hosp Community Psychiatry 35(8):813–820, 1984

Jones SL, Dimond M: Family theory and family therapy models: comparative review with implications for nursing practice. J Psychosoc Nurs Ment Health Serv 20(10):12–19, 1982

Myers JK et al: Six-month prevalence of psychiatric disorders in three communities, 1980–1982. Arch Gen Psychiatry 41(10):959–967, 1984

Nadi NS, Nurnberger JI, Gershon ES: Muscarinic cholinergic receptors on skin fibroblasts in familial affective disorder. N Engl J Med 311(4):225–230, 1984

Uhlenhuth EH et al: Symptom checklist syndromes in the general population. Arch Gen Psychiatry 40(11):167–173, 1983

Pamphlets

Witkin MJ: Trends in Patient Care Episodes in Mental Health Facilities, 1955–1977. Mental Health Statistical Note No. 154. US Department of Health and Human Services, September, 1980

THERAPEUTIC RELATIONSHIP

Books

Bradley J, Edinberg M: Communication in the Nursing Context. New York, Appleton-Century-Crofts, 1982

Bridge W, Clark J (eds): Communication in Nursing Care. London, HM & M Publishers, 1981

Carkhuff R: Helping and Human Relations: Practice and Research. New York, Holt, Rinehart, & Winston, 1969

Collins M: Communication in Health Care: The Human Connection in the Life Cycle. St Louis, CV Mosby, 1983

Danziger K: Interpersonal Communication. New York, Pergamon Press, 1976

Duldt B, Giffin K, Patton B: Interpersonal Communication in Nursing. Philadelphia, FA Davis, 1984

Edwards B, Brilhart J: Communication in Nursing Practice. St Louis, CV Mosby, 1981

Fromm-Reichmann F: Principles of Intensive Psychotherapy. Chicago, University of Chicago Press, 1971

Hammond D, Hepworth D, Smith V: Improving Therapeutic Communication. San Francisco, Jossey-Bass, 1977

Hein E: Communication in Nursing Practice. Boston, Little, Brown, 1980

Kim M, McFarland G, McLane A (eds): Classification of Nursing Diagnoses: Proceedings of the Fifth National Conference. St Louis, CV Mosby, 1984

Kim M, McFarland G, McLane A: Pocket Guide to Nursing Diagnoses. St Louis, CV Mosby, 1984

Lewis G: Nurse–Patient Communication. Dubuque, Wm C Brown, 1978

McFarland G, Leonard H, Morris M: Nursing Leadership and Management: Contemporary Strategies. New York, John Wiley, 1984

Murphy C, Hunter H: Ethical Problems in the Nurse–Patient Relationship. Boston, Allyn & Bacon, 1983

O'Brien M: Communications and Relationships in Nursing. St Louis, CV Mosby, 1978

Peplau H: Basic Principles of Patient Counseling. Philadelphia, Smith, Kline, & French Laboratories, 1964

Pluckhan M: Human Communication: The Matrix of Nursing. New York, McGraw-Hill, 1978

Purtilo R: Health Professional–Patient Interaction. Philadephia, WB Saunders, 1978

Ruesch J: Therapeutic Communication. New York, WW Norton, 1973

Ruesch J: Communication and psychiatry. In Kaplan H, Freedman A, Sadock B (eds): Comprehensive Textbook of Psychiatry, vol. 1. Baltimore, Williams and Wilkins, 1980

Sierra-Franco M: Therapeutic Communications in Nursing. New York, McGraw-Hill, 1978

Springer S, Deutsch G: Left Brain, Right Brain. San Francisco, WH Freeman, 1981

Sundeen S, Stuart G, Rankin E, Cohen S: Nurse–Client Interaction: Implementing the Nursing Process. St Louis, CV Mosby, 1981

Topalis M, Aguilera D: Psychiatric Nursing. St Louis, CV Mosby, 1978

Truax C, Carkhuff R: Toward Effective Counseling and Psychotherapy: Training and Practice. Chicago, Aldine-Atherton, 1967

Watzlawick P, Beavin J, Jackson D: Pragmatics of Human Communication. New York, WW Norton, 1967

Wiedenbach E, Falls C: Communication, Key to Effective Nursing. New York, Tiresias Press, 1978

Wilson H, Kneisl C: Psychiatric Nursing. Menlo Park, CA, Addison-Wesley, 1979

Articles

Almore M: Dyadic communication. Am J Nurs 79(6):1076–1078, 1979

Authier J, Authier K, Lutey M: Clinical management of the tearfully depressed patient: communication skills for the nurse practitioner. J Psychiatr Nurs 17(2):34–41, 1979

Blount M, Green S, Hamory A et al: Documenting with the problem-oriented record system. Am J Nurs 78(9):1539–1542, 1978

Boettcher E: Nurse-client collaboration: dynamic equilibrium in the nursing care system. J Psychiatr Nurs 16(12):7–15, 1978

Brink T: Is TLC contraindicated for geriatric patients? Perspect Psychiatr Care 15(3):129–131, 1977

Brockopp D: What is NLP? Am J Nurs 83(7):1012–1014, 1983

Carser D, Doona M: Alienation: A nursing concept. J Psychiatr Nurs 16(9):33–40, 1978

Cosper B: How well do patients understand hospital jargon? Am J Nurs 77(12):1932–1934, 1977

Daubenmire M, Searles S, Ashton C: A methodologic framework to study nurse–patient communication. Nurs Res 27(5):303–310, 1978

Doona M, Annino S, Kelleher M: Professional affirmation in nursing care. J Psychiatr Nurs 15(8):16–23, 1977

Fahrner B, Ellis N, Stark S et al: Record-keeping in a state hospital: a modification of the Weed system. Hosp Commun Psychiatry 28(12):907–908, 1977

Frenkel S, Greden J, Robinson J et al: Does patient contact change racial perceptions? Am J Nurs 80(7):1340–1342, 1980

Gagan J: Methodological notes on empathy. ANS 5(2):65–72, 1983

Giffords, Maberry D: An integrated system for computerized patient records. Hosp Commun Psychiatry 30(8):532–535, 1979

Gluck J: The computerized medical record system; meeting the challenge for nursing. J Nurs Admin 9(12):17–24, 1979

Hall B: The effect of interpersonal attraction on the therapeutic relationship: a review and suggestions for further study. J Psychiatr Nurs 15(9):18–23, 1977

Hardin S, Halaris A: Nonverbal communication of patients and high and low empathy nurses. J Psychosoc Nurs 21(1):14–19, 1983

Heineken J: Disconfirmation in dysfunctional communication. Nurs Res 31(4): 211–213, 1982

Heineken J: Treating the disconfirmed psychiatric client. J Psychosoc Nurs 21(1):21–25, 1983

Johnson M: Self-disclosure: a variable in the nurse-client relationship. J Psychiatr Nurs 18(1):17–20, 1980

Kalisch B: What is empathy? Am J Nurs 73(9):1548–1552, 1973

Kaplan N, Levy K: An approach for facilitating the passage through termination. J Psychiatr Nurs 16(6):11–14, 1978

Karns P, Schwab T: Therapeutic communication and clinical instruction. Nurs Outlook 30(1):39–43, 1982

Karshmer J, Kornfeld-Jacobs G, Carr A: Causal attributions: bias in the nurse-patient relationship. J Psychiatr Nurs 18(5):25–30, 1980

Kasch C: Interpersonal competence and communication in the delivery of nursing care. ANS 6(2):71–88, 1984

Kauffman M: On developing empathy; sharing the patient's experience. Am J Nurs 78(5):860–861, 1978

Knowles R: Thorough neuro-linguistic programming. Am J Nurs 83(7):1011–1014, 1983

Krikorian D, Paulanka B: Self-awareness—The key to a successful nurse–patient relationship? J Psychosoc Nurs 20(6):19–21, 1982

Lego S: The one-to-one nurse–patient relationship. Perspect Psychiatr Care 18(2):67–89, 1980

Littlefield N: Therapeutic relationship: a brief encounter. Am J Nurs 82(9):1395–1399, 1982

McCann J: Termination of the psychotherapeutic relationship. J Psychiatr Nurs 17(10):37–46, 1979

McFarland G, Apostoles F: The nursing history in a psychiatric setting: adaptations to a variety of nursing care patterns and patient populations. J Psychiatr Nurs 13(4):12–17, 1975

McNeill D: Developing the complete computer-based information system. J Nurs Adm 9(11):34–46, 1979

Pelletier L: Interpersonal communications task group. J Psychosoc Nurs 21(9):33–36, 1983

Ramaekers M: Communication blocks revisited. Am J Nurs 79(6):1079–1081, 1979

Rawnsley M: Toward a conceptual base for affective nursing. Nurs Outlook 28(4):244–247, 1980

Ricci M. An experiment with personal-space invasion in the nurse–patient relationship and its effect on anxiety. Issues Ment Health Nurs 3(3):203–218, 1981

Rieder K, Wood M: Problem-orientation: an experimental study to test its heuristic value. Nurs Res 27(1):25–29, 1978

Ruditis S: Developing trust in nursing interpersonal relationships. J Psychiatr Nurs 17(4):20–23, 1979

Scheideman J: Problem patients do not exist. Am J Nurs 79(6):1082–1084, 1979

Seeger P: Self-awareness and nursing. J Psychiatr Nurs 15(8):24–26, 1977

Sharkey P, Lipshutz M: Nursing care of the mentally retarded: communication issues. Issues Ment Health Nurs 4(3):191–197, 1982

Sparling S, Jones S: Setting: a contextual variable associated with empathy. J Psychiatr Nurs 15(4):9–12, 1977

Swearingen D, Messick J, May P et al: Improving patient care through measurement: goal importance and achievement scaling. J Psychiatr Nurs 15(9):30–36, 1977

Topf M, Damacher B: Predominant source of interpersonal influence in relationships between psychiatric patients and nursing staff. Res Nurs Health 2(1):35–43, 1979

Topf M, Dambacher B: Teaching interpersonal skills: a model for facilitating optimal interpersonal relations. J Psychosoc Nurs 19(12):29–33, 1981

Wallston K, Cohen B, Wallston B et al: Increasing nurses' person-centeredness. Nurs Res 27(3):156–159, 1978

Wlody G: Effective communication techniques. Nurs Manage 12(10):19–22, 1981

Wyatt M, Withersty D: Teaching interpersonal management for effective professional nursing practice. J Psychiatr Nurs 17(6):23–27, 1979

PSYCHIATRIC ASSESSMENT OF THE ADULT

Books

Arieti S (ed): American Handbook of Psychiatry, vol 1. New York, Basic Books, 1974

Butler R, and Lewis M: Aging and Mental Health: Positive Psychosocial Approaches. St Louis, CV Mosby, 1977

Diagnostic and Statistical Manual of Mental Disorders, 3rd ed. Washington DC, The American Psychiatric Association, 1980

Division of Psychiatric and Mental Health Nursing Practice. Standards of Psychiatric and Mental Health Nursing Practice. Kansas City, The American Nurses Association, 1982

Freedman A, Kaplan H, Sadock B: Modern Synopsis of Comprehensive Textbook of Psychiatry II. Baltimore, Williams & Wilkins, 1978

Goble F: The Third Force. New York, Grossman Publishers, 1975

Kim M, McFarland G, McLane A: Classification of Nursing Diagnoses: Proceedings of the Fifth National Conference. St Louis, CV Mosby, 1984

Kim M, McFarland G, McLane A: Pocket Guide to Nursing Diagnoses. St Louis, CV Mosby, 1984

Kim M, Moritz D: Classification of Nursing Diagnoses. Proceedings of Third and Fourth National Conference. New York, McGraw-Hill, 1982

Kolb L: Modern Clinical Psychiatry, 10th ed. Philadelphia, WB Saunders, 1982

Manfreda M, Krampitz S: Psychiatric Nursing. Philadelphia, FA Davis, 1977

Maslow A: Toward a Psychology of Being. New York, Van Nostrand Reinhold, 1968

Meldman M, McFarland G, Johnson E: The Problem-Oriented Psychiatric Index and Treatment Plans. St Louis, CV Mosby, 1976

Nicholi A (ed): The Harvard Guide to Modern Psychiatry. Cambridge, Harvard University Press, 1978

Orem D: Nursing: Concepts of Practice, 3rd ed. New York, McGraw-Hill, 1985

Reid W, Balis G, Donaldson J: Treatment of the DSM-III Psychiatric Disorders. New York, Brunner/Mazel Publishers, 1983

Riehl J, Roy C: Conceptual Models for Nursing Practice. New York, Appleton-Century-Crofts, 1974

Articles

Bumbalo J, Siemon M: Nursing assessment and diagnosis: mental health problems of children. Top Clin Nurs 5(1):41–54, 1983

Bridge P, Carlson R: Preadmission assessment of the elderly. Can Nurse 79(11):27–29, 1983

Carmack B: Guidelines for assessing mental/psychosocial status. Occup Health Nurs 30(5):29–34, 1982

Cohen S: Mental status assessment. Am J Nurs 81(8):1493–1518, 1981

Craig T, Goodman A, Haugland G: Impact of DSM-III on clinical practice. Am J Psychiatry 139(7):922–925, 1982

Dodd M. Assessing mental status. Am J Nurs 78(9):1501–1503, 1978

Falcioni D: Assessing the abused elderly. J Gerontol Nurs 8:208–212, 1982

Goldenberg B et al: Assessing behavior: The nurse's mental status exam. Geriatr Nurs 5(2):94–98, 1984

Green N: A psychiatric assessment tool for staff and students. J Psychiatr Nurs 17(4):28–31, 1979

Guthrie D: Psychosocial side of diabetes and its complications. Diabetes Educator 8:24–28, 1982

Hill L et al: Client assessment: an integrated model. J Nurs Educ 20:16–23, 1981

Kleh J, Lange P, Karu E et al: Differential diagnosis of the disturbed elderly patient. Hosp Community Psychiatry 29(11):735–738, 1978

Mackenzie T, Popkin M, Callies A: Clinical applications of DSM-III in consultation-liaison psychiatry. Hosp Community Psychiatry 34(7):628–633, 1983

Malt U: Classification and diagnosis of depression. ACTA Psychiatrica Scandinavica Supplementum 67(302):7–30, 1983

Mawson D: Organic psychiatric disorders. Assessment of the mental state. Nurs Times 79(24):41–42, 1983

McFarland G, Apostoles F: The nursing history in a psychiatric setting: adaptations to a variety of nursing care patterns and patient populations. J Psychiatr Nurs 13:12–17, 1975

McKegney F, McMahon T, King J: The use of DSM-III in a general hospital consultation-liaison service. Gen Hosp Psychiatry 5(2):115–121, 1983

Mezzich J, Coffman G, Goodpastor S: Format for DSM-III diagnostic formulation: experience with 1,111 consecutive patients. Am J Psychiatry 139(5):591–596, 1982

Millon T: The DSM-III: an insider's perspective. Am Psychol 38(7):804–814, 1983

Morgan S, Macey M: Three assessment tools for family therapy. J Psychiatr Nurs 16(3):39–42, 1978

Natapoff J, Moetzinger C, Quarto J: Health assessment skills in the baccalaureate program. Nurs Outlook 30(1):44–47, 1982

Pepper J: Psychiatric assessment on a forensic unit. Can Nurse 78:50–51, 1982

Reynolds J, Logsdon J: Assessing your patient's mental status. Nursing '79 9(8)26–33, 1979

Silverstein M, Warren R, Harrow M, et al: Changes in diagnosis from DSM-II to the research diagnostic criteria and DSM-III. Am J Psychiatry 139(3):366–368, 1982

Skodol A, Spitzer R: DSM-III: rationale, basic concepts, and some differences from ICD-9. Acta Psychiatr Scand 66(4):271–281, 1982

Spitzer R, Skodol A, Williams J, et al: Supervising intake diagnosis. Arch Gen Psychiatry 39(11):1299–1305, 1982

Stein M, Willick M: Clinical aspects of character. J Am Psychoanal Assoc 31(1):225–236, 1983

Talley S: Data collection methods. Psychiatric vs. psychosocial concepts. Nurse Pract 8(5):83–85, 1983

Taylor P: The elements of a comprehensive mental health assessment. Can J Psychiatr Nurs 24(2):12–15, 1983

Tripp-Reimer T, Brink P, Saunders J: Cultural assessment: content and process. Nurs Outlook 32(2):78–82, 1984

Whitley M, Willingham D: Adding a sexual assessment to the health interview. J Psychiatr Nurs 16(4):17, 22–27, 1978

Williams J et al: A psychiatric nursing perspective on DSM-III . . . Diagnostic and Statistical Manual of Mental Disorders. J Psychosoc Nurs 20(4):14–20, 1982

Wulach J: Diagnosing the DSM-III antisocial personality disorder. Prof Psychol Res Pract 14(3):330–349, 1983

Unpublished Material

Nursing Education Section. Conceptual framework. Washington DC, St. Elizabeths Hospital, 1979

NURSING DIAGNOSES IN CARING FOR THE PSYCHIATRIC PATIENT
General

Books

American Psychiatric Association: Diagnostic and Statistical Manual of Mental Disorders, 3rd ed. Washington DC, American Psychiatric Association, 1980

Beck C, Rawlins R, Williams S (eds): Mental Health–Psychiatric Nursing: A Holistic Life-Cycle Approach. St Louis, CV Mosby, 1984

Doona M: Travelbee's Intervention in Psychiatric Nursing, 2nd ed. Philadelphia, FA Davis, 1979

Gebbie K: Summary of the Second National Conference—Classification of Nursing Diagnoses. St Louis, The Clearinghouse, St Louis University, 1976

Haber J, Leach AM, Schudy SM, Sideleau BF (eds): Comprehensive Psychiatric Nursing. New York, McGraw-Hill, 1982

Hagerty B: Psychiatric-Mental Health Assessment. St Louis, CV Mosby, 1984.

Joel L, Collins D: Psychiatric Nursing Theory and Application. New York, McGraw-Hill, 1978

Kalkman M, Davis A: New Dimensions in Mental Health—Psychiatric Nursing, 5th ed. New York, McGraw-Hill, 1980

Kim M, McFarland G, McLane A (eds): Classification of Nursing Diagnoses: Proceedings of the Fifth National Conference. St Louis, CV Mosby, 1984

Kim M, McFarland G, McLane A (eds): Pocket Guide to Nursing Diagnoses. St Louis, CV Mosby, 1984

Koldjeski D: Community Mental Health Nursing: New Directions in Theory and Practice. New York, John Wiley & Sons, 1984

Kreigh H, Perko J: Psychiatric–Mental Health Nursing: A Commitment to Care and Concern. Reston, Reston Publishing, 1979

Kyes J, Hofling CK: Basic Psychiatric Concepts in Nursing, 4th ed. Philadelphia, JB Lippincott, 1980

Madden J: A Guide to Alcohol and Drug Dependence. Bristol, John Wright & Sons, 1979

McFarland G, Leonard H, Morris M: Nursing Leadership and Management: Contemporary Strategies. New York, John Wiley & Sons, 1984

Meldman M, McFarland G, Johnson E: The Problem-Oriented Psychiatric Index and Treatment Plans. St Louis, CV Mosby, 1976

Murray R, Huelskoetter M: Psychiatric Mental Health Nursing: Giving Emotional Care. Englewood Cliffs, NJ, Prentice-Hall, 1983

Pasquali E, Alesi E, Arnold H, De Basio N: Mental Health Nursing: A Bio-Psycho-Cultural Approach. St Louis, CV Mosby, 1981

Robinson L: Psychiatric Nursing as a Human Experience. Philadelphia, WB Saunders, 1983

Stuart GW, Sundeen SJ: Principles and Practice of Psychiatric Nursing. St Louis, CV Mosby, 1983

Taylor C: Mereness' Essentials of Psychiatric Nursing. St Louis, CV Mosby, 1982

Topalis M, Aguilera D: Psychiatric Nursing, 7th ed. St Louis, CV Mosby, 1978

Wilson HS, Kneisl CR: Psychiatric Nursing. Menlo Park, CA, Addison-Wesley Publishing, 1983

Nursing Diagnoses

Books

Campbell C: Nursing Diagnosis and Intervention in Nursing Practice. New York, John Wiley & Sons, 1984

Carpenito L: Nursing Diagnoses: Application to Clinical Practice. Philadelphia, JB Lippincott, 1983

Douglas D, Murphy E: Nursing process, nursing diagnoses, and emerging taxonomies. In J McClosky, H Grace (eds): Current Issues in Nursing. Boston, Blackwell Scientific Publications, 1981

Gebbie K: Summary of the Second National Conference—Classification of Nursing Diagnoses. St Louis, The Clearinghouse, St Louis University, 1976

Gebbie K, Lavin M (eds): Classification of Nursing Diagnoses. St Louis, CV Mosby, 1975

Gordon M: Nursing Diagnosis: Process and Application. New York, McGraw-Hill, 1982

Kim M, McFarland G, McLane A: Classification of Nursing Diagnoses: Proceedings of the Fifth National Conference. St Louis, CV Mosby, 1984

Kim M, McFarland G, McLane A: Pocket Guide to Nursing Diagnoses. St Louis, CV Mosby, 1984

Kim M, Moritz D: Classification of Nursing Diagnoses: Proceedings of Third and Fourth National Conference. New York, McGraw-Hill, 1981

Lash A: Nursing diagnoses: some comments on the gap between theory and practice. In J McClosky, H Grace (eds): Current Issues in Nursing. Boston, Blackwell Scientific Publications, 1981

Soares C: Nursing and medical diagnoses: A comparison of variant and essential features. In Chaska N (ed): The Nursing Profession: Views Through the Mist. New York, McGraw-Hill, 1978

Articles

Bircher A: On the development and classification of diagnoses. Nurs Forum 14(1):10–29, 1975

Bruce J: Implementation of nursing diagnosis: A nursing administrator's perspective. Nurs Clin North Am 14(3):509–515, 1979

Dossey B, Guzzetta C: Nursing diagnoses: How to define the problem can be half the solution. Nursing '81 11(6):34, 1981

Fortin J, Rabinow J: Legal implications of nursing diagnosis. Nurs Clin North Am 14(3):553–561, 1979

Fredette S, Gloriant F: Nursing diagnosis in cancer chemotherapy: in practice. Am J Nurs 81:2021, 1981

Fredette S, Gloriant F: Nursing diagnosis in cancer chemotherapy: in theory. Am J Nurs 81:2013, 1981

Fredette S, O'Connor K: Nursing diagnosis in teaching and curriculum planning. Nurs Clin North Am 14(3):541–552, 1979

Gebbie K, Lavin M: Classifying nursing diagnoses. Am J Nurs 74(2):250–253, 1974

Gleit C, Tatro S: Nursing diagnosis for healthy individuals. Nurs Health Care 2:456, 1981

Gordon M: Nursing diagnoses and the diagnostic process. Am J Nurs 76(8):1298–1300, 1976

Gordon M: The concept of nursing diagnosis. Nurs Clin North Am 14(3):487–495, 1979

Gordon M: Determining study topics. Nurs Res 29:83, 1980

Gordon M: Predictive strategies in diagnostic tasks. Nurs Res 29(1):39–45, 1980

Gordon M, Sweeney M: Methodological problems and issues in identifying and standardizing nursing diagnoses. Adv Nurs Sc 2(1):1–15, 1979

Guzzetta C, Forsyth G: Nursing diagnostic pilot study: psychophysiologic stress. Adv Nurs Sc 2(1):27–44, 1979

Hausman K: The concept and application of nursing diagnosis. J Neurosurg Nurs 12(2):76, 1980

Jones P, Jakob D: Nursing diagnosis: differentiating fear and anxiety. Nurs Papers (Can) 13(4):20, 1981

Leslie F: Nursing diagnosis: Use in long-term care. Am J Nurs 81:1012, 1981

Loomis M, Wood D: Cure: The potential outcome of nursing care. Image 15:4, 1983

Lunney M: Nursing diagnosis: refining the system. Am J Nurs 82:456, 1982

McFarland G, Naschinski C: Impaired communication—a descriptive study. Nurs Clin North Am, 20(4):775–785, 1985

Mundinger M, Jauron G: Developing a nursing diagnosis. Nurs Outlook 23(2):94–98, 1975

Perry A: Nursing diagnosis research. J Neurosurg Nurs 14(2):108, 1982

Popkess S: Diagnosing your patient's strengths. Nursing '81 11(7):34, 1981

Price M: Nursing diagnosis: making a concept come alive. Am J Nurs 80:668, 1980

Roberts C: Identifying the real patient problems. Nurs Clin North Am 17:481, 1982

Roy C: A diagnostic classification system for nursing. Nurs Outlook 23(2):90–94, 1975

Shoemaker J: How nursing diagnosis helps focus your care. RN 42(8):56–61, 1979

Weber S: Nursing diagnosis in private practice. Nurs Clin North Am 14(3):533–539, 1979

Unpublished Material

Task Force of the National Group for the Classification of Nursing Diagnoses: Subcommittee Report on Definition of Nursing Diagnoses. The Fourth National Conference on Classification of Nursing Diagnoses, St Louis, April 9–13, 1980

Aggression, Inappropriate

Books

Bandura A: Aggression: A Social Learning Analysis. Englewood Cliffs, NJ, Prentice-Hall, 1973

Blake K, Taylor C: The Prevention and Management of Aggressive Behavior. Columbia, SC, Department of Mental Health, 1977

Brain P, Benton D (eds): Multidisciplinary Approaches to Aggression. New York, Bio-Medical Press, 1981

Crabtree J, Moyer K: Bibliography of Aggressive Behavior. New York, Liss, 1981

Edmunds G, Kendrick D: The Measurement of Human Aggressiveness. New York, John Wiley & Sons, 1980

Fawcett J (ed): Dynamics of Violence. Chicago, American Medical Association, 1971

Geen R, Donnerstein E (eds): Aggression: Theoretical and Methodological Issues. New York, Academic Press, 1981

Geen R, Donnerstein E (eds): Aggression, Theoretical, and Empirical Reviews. New York, Academic Press, 1983

Goldstein A: In Response to Aggression: Methods of Control and Prosocial Alternative. New York, Pergamon Press, 1981

Goldstein A: Prevention and Control of Aggression. New York, Pergamon Press, 1983

Gottheil E (ed): Alcohol, Drug Abuse, and Aggression. Springfield, IL, Charles C Thomas, 1983

Hamburg D, Trudeau M (eds): Biobehavioral Aspects of Aggression. New York, Liss, 1981

Lathrop VG: The client with homicidal behavior. In Gorton JG, Partridge R (eds): Practice and Management of Psychiatric Emergency Care. St Louis, CV Mosby, 1982

Lion J: Evaluation and Management of the Violent Patient. Springfield, IL, Charles C Thomas, 1972

Lion J, Reid W: Assault Within Psychiatric Facilities. New York, Grune & Stratton, 1983

Simmel E, Hahn M, Walters J (eds): Aggressive Behavior, Genetic and Neural Approaches. Hillsdale, NY, Lawrence Erlbaum, 1983

Stegne L: The Prevention and Management of Disturbed Behavior. Toronto, Ontario Government Book Store, 1977

Valzelli L: Psychobiology of Aggression and Violence. New York, Raven Press, 1981

Zarfas D, Goldberg B (eds): Aggression, Mental Illness, Mental Retardation: Psychobiological Approaches. London, Ontario, University of Western Ontario, 1980

Zillman D: Connections Between Sex and Aggression. Hillsdale, NY, Lawrence Erlbaum, 1983

Articles

Anderson D: The relationships among assertion, aggression, and anxiety (doctoral dissertation, University of South Florida, 1981). Dissertation Abstracts International 41(10-B):3878, 1981

Armstrong B: Conference report. Handling the violent patient in the hospital. Hosp Community Psychiatry 29(7):463–467, 1978

Berry P: DRO: Practical applications to reduce aggressive and disruptive behavior. Can J Psychiatr Nurs 23:16–18, 1982

Boyd W: Communication tactics for neutralizing verbal aggression (doctoral dissertation, Washington State University, 1982). Dissertation Abstracts International 43(2-A):305, 1982

Brigman C, Dickey C, Zegeer L: The agitated aggressive patient. Am J Nurs 83(10):1409–1412, 1983

Buikhuisen W: Aggressive behavior and cognitive disorders. Int J Law Psychiatry 5(2):205–217, 1982

Bursten B: Using mechanical restraints on acutely disturbed psychiatric patients. Hosp Community Psychiatry 26(11): 757–758, 1975

Buss A, Durkee A: An inventory for assessing different kinds of hostility. J Consult Psychol 21(4):343–349, 1957

Campbell M, Cohen I, Small A: Drugs in aggressive behavior. J Am Acad Child Psychiatry 21(2):107–117, 1982

Cocozza J, Steadman H: Some refinements in the measurement and prediction of dangerous behavior. Am J Psychiatry 131(9):1012–1014, 1974

Cooper S, Browne F, McClean K, King D: Aggressive behavior in a psychiatric observation ward. Acta Psychiatr Scand 68(5):386–393, 1983

Driscoll J: Perception of an aggressive interaction as a function of the perceiver's aggression. Percept Mot Skills 54:1123–1134, 1982

Edelman S: Managing the violent patient in a community mental health center. Hosp Community Psychiatry 29(7):460–462, 1978

Gutheil T: Observations on the theoretical basis for seclusion of the psychiatric inpatient. Am J Psychiatry 135(3):325–328, 1978

Harrington J: Violence: a clinical viewpoint. Br Med J 1(5794):228–231, 1982

Holm O: Four factors affecting perceived aggressiveness. J Psychology 114:227–234, 1983

Karhmer J: The application of social learning theory to aggression. Perspect Psychiatr Care 16(5–6):223–227, 1978

Kettlewell P, Kausch D: The generalization of the effects of a cognitive-behavioral treatment program for aggressive children. J Abnorm Child Psychol 11(1):101–114, 1983

Lambert W: Toward an integrative theory of children's aggression. Ital J Psychol 8(2):153–164, 1981

Lanza M: Origins of aggression. J Psychosoc Nurs Ment Health Serv 21(6):11–16, 1983

Lathrop V: Aggression as a response. Perspect Psychiatr Care 16(5–6):202–205, 1978

Lenefsky B, dePalma T, Locicero D: Management of violent behaviors. Perspect Psychiatr Care 16(5–6):212–217, 1978

Maynard C, Chitty K: Dealing with anger: guidelines for nursing intervention. J Psychiatr Nurs 17(6):36–41, 1979

Moos R: Size, staffing, and psychiatric ward treatment environments. Arch Gen Psychiatry 26(5):414–418, 1972

Moritz D: Understanding anger. Am J Nurs 78(1):81–83, 1978

Munn T: The meaning and experience of aggression in middle adolescence: a phenomenological approach (doctoral dissertation, California School of Professional Psychology, 1982). Dissertation Abstracts International 43(3-B):915, 1982

Murphy P, Schultz E: Passive-aggressive behavior in patients and staff. J Psychiatr Nurs 16(3):43–45, 1978

Nichtern S: The sociocultural and psychodynamic aspects of the acting-out and violent adolescent. Adolesc Psychiatry 10:140–146, 1982

Penningroth P: Control of violence in a mental health setting. Am J Nurs 75(4):606–609, 1975

Perry R: Modeling and token reinforcement in the reduction of children's aggression (doctoral dissertation, Arizona State University, 1981). Dissertation Abstracts International 41 (10-B): 3901, 1981

Reese D: Perceptions of family social climate and physical aggression in the home (doctoral dissertation, University of South Dakota, 1982). Dissertation Abstracts International 42 (12-B):4939, 1982

Ruby N: Personal space and the perception of assertion versus aggression (doctoral dissertation, University of South Dakota, 1983). Dissertation Abstracts International 43(10-B):3374, 1983

Rumpler C, Seigerman C: A behavior modification approach to dealing with violent behavior in an Intensive Care Unit. Perspect Psychiatr Care 16(5–6):206–211; 245, 1978

Sadowski C, Wenzel D: The relationship of locus of control dimensions to reported hostility and aggression. J Psychol 112(2):227–230, 1982

Slife B, Rychlak J: Role of affective assessment in modeling aggressive behavior. J Perspect Soc Psychol 43(4):461–468, 1982

Smith K: Effect of patient management training on nursing intervention in aggressive behavior: An evaluative study (doctoral dissertation, North Carolina State University, 1983). Dissertation Abstracts International 43(12-A):3784, 1983

Spotnitz H: Aggression in the therapy of schizophrenia. Mod Psychoanal 6(2):131–140, 1981

Stewart A: Handling the aggressive patient. Perspect Psychiatr Care 16(5–6):228–232, 1978

Tardiff K: The use of medication for assaultive patients. Hosp Community Psychiatry 33(4):307–308, 1982

Warren R, Kurlychek R: Treatment of maladaptive anger and aggression. Catharsis vs. behavior therapy. J Behav Technol Meth Ther 27(3):135–139, 1981

Anxiety: Mild, Moderate, Severe, Extreme (Panic)

Books

Burrows G, Davies B (eds): Handbook of Studies on Anxiety. Amsterdam, Elsevier/North Holland Biomedical Press, 1980

Jones P, Jacob D: Anxiety revisited—From a practice perspective. In Kim M, McFarland G, McLane A (eds): Classification of Nursing Diagnoses: Proceedings of the Fifth National Conference. St Louis, CV Mosby, 1984

Kalkman M, Davis A: New Dimensions in Mental Health–Psychiatric Nursing. New York, McGraw-Hill, 1980

Kaplan H, Freedman A, Sadock B: Comprehensive Textbook of Psychiatry. Baltimore, Williams & Wilkins, 1980

Kelly D: Anxiety and Emotions. Springfield, IL, Charles C Thomas, 1980

Kim M, McFarland G, McLane A: Pocket Guide to Nursing Diagnoses. St Louis, CV Mosby, 1984

Klein D: Anxiety reconceptualized. In Klein D, Rabkin J: Anxiety: New Research and Changing Concepts. New York, Raven Press, 1981

May R: The Meaning of Anxiety. New York, W Norton, 1977

McFarland G, Wasli E: Mild anxiety, moderate anxiety, severe anxiety, extreme anxiety (panic). In Kim M, McFarland G, McLane A (eds): Pocket Guide to Nursing Diagnoses. St Louis, CV Mosby, 1984

Meldman M, McFarland G, Johnson E: The Problem-Oriented Psychiatric Index and Treatment Plans. St Louis, CV Mosby, 1976

Peplau H: A working definition of anxiety. In Burd S, Marshall M (eds): Some Clinical Approaches to Psychiatric Nursing. New York, Macmillan, 1966

Sarason I, Spielberger C (eds): Stress and Anxiety, Vol 7. New York, Hemisphere Publishing, 1980

Spielberger C, Sarason I, Milgram N (eds): Stress and Anxiety, Vol. 8. New York, Hemisphere Publishing, 1982

Yocom C: The differentiation of fear and anxiety. In Kim M, McFarland G, McLane A (eds): Classification of Nursing Diagnoses: Proceedings of the Fifth National Conference. St Louis, CV Mosby, 1984

Articles

Archer R, Kutash K: Anxiety response to psychological feedback among psychiatric inpatients. Psychol Rep 50:547–551, 1982

Highland A: Anxiety: A summary of past and present research and theory. Child Welfare 60(8):519–528, 1981

Holderby R, McNulty E: Feelings feelings. Nursing '79 9(10):39–43, 1979

Johnston M: Recognition of patients' worries by nurses and by other patients. Br J Clin Psych 21:255–261, 1982

Johnston M, Carpenter L: Relationship between preoperative anxiety and postoperative state. Psychol Med 10:361–367, 1980

Kerr N: Anxiety: Theoretical considerations. Perspect Psychiatr Care 16(1):36–40; 46, 1978

Knowles R: Dealing with feelings: managing anxiety. Am J Nurs 81(1):110–111, 1981

Kristic J: Anxiety levels of hospitalized psychiatric patients throughout total hospitalization. J Psychiatr Nurs 17(7):33–34; 37–42, 1979

Liebowitz M, Klein D: Case 1, Assessment and treatment of phobic anxiety. J Clin Psychol 40(11):486–492, 1979

Pfeiffer E: Handling the distressed older patient. Geriatrics 34(2):24–25; 28–29, 1979

Ricci M: An experiment with personal-space invasion in the nurse–patient relationship and its effect on anxiety. Issues Ment Health Nurs 3:203–218, 1981

Communication, Impaired

Books

Berne E: Games People Play. The Psychology of Human Relationships. New York, Grove Press, 1966

Berne E: What Do You Say After You Say Hello? New York, Bantam Books, 1973
Bradley J, Edinberg M: Communication in the Nursing Context. New York, Appleton-Century-Crofts, 1982
Bridge W, Clark J (ed): Communication in Nursing Care. London, HM & M, 1981
Ceccio J, Ceccio C: Effective Communication in Nursing: Theory and Practice. New York, John Wiley & Sons, 1982
Duldt B, Giffin K, Patton B: Interpersonal Communication in Nursing. Philadelphia, FA Davis, 1983
Edwards B, Brilhart J: Communication in Nursing Practice. St Louis, CV Mosby, 1981
Gazda G, Childers W, Walters R: Interpersonal Communication: A Handbook for Health Professionals. Rockville, MD, Aspen Systems Corp, 1982
Haber J, Leach A, Schudy, S, Sideau B: Comprehensive Psychiatric Nursing. New York, McGraw-Hill, 1982
Hein E: Communication in Nursing Practice. Boston, Little, Brown, 1980
Kim M, McFarland G, McLane A: Pocket Guide to Nursing Diagnoses. St Louis, CV Mosby, 1984
McFarland G, Leonard H, Morris M: Nursing Leadership and Management: Contemporary Strategies. New York, John Wiley & Sons, 1984
Ruesch J: Communication and psychiatry. In Kaplan H, Freedman A, Sadock B (eds): Comprehensive Textbook of Psychiatry. Baltimore, Williams & Wilkins, 1980
Ruesch J: Disturbed Communication; The Clinical Assessment of Normal and Pathological Communication Behavior. New York, WW Norton, 1972
Satir V: Conjoint Family Therapy. Palo Alto, CA, Science and Behavior Books, 1967
Shanks S (ed): Nursing and the Management of Adult Communication Disorders. San Diego, College-Hill Press, 1983
Shanks S (ed): Nursing and the Management of Pediatric Communication Disorders. San Diego, College-Hill Press, 1983
Springer S, Deutsch G: Left Brain, Right Brain. San Francisco, WH Freeman, 1981
Watzlawick P, Beavin J, Jackson D: Pragmatics of Human Communication. New York, WW Norton, 1967

Articles

Bashor P: A nursing communication assessment guide. Rehab Nurs 8(1):20–21; 30, 1983
Hardin S, Halaris A: Nonverbal communication of patients and high and low empathy nurses. J Psychiatr Nurs Ment Health Serv 21(1):14–19, 1983
Heidt P: Effect of therapeutic touch on anxiety level of hospitalized patients. Nurs Res 30:32–37, 1981
Heineken J: Treating the disconfirmed psychiatric client. J Psychiatr Nurs Ment Health Serv 21(1):21–25, 1983
Henrich A, Bernheim K: Responding to patient's concerns. Nurs Outlook 29:428–433, 1981
MacKay R: Hearing and responding: communicating with the critically ill. Dimens Health Serv 58(8):18–19, 1981
Scott D, Oberst M, Dropkin M: A stress-coping model. Adv Nurs Sci 95(2):99–108, 1980

Unpublished Material

Sieburg E: Dysfunctional Communication and Interpersonal Responsiveness in Small Groups. Unpublished Doctoral Dissertation, University of Denver, 1969

Coping, Ineffective Individual

Books

Cameron R, Meichenbaum D: The nature of effective coping and the treatment of stress related problems: a cognitive-behavioral perspective. In Goldberger L and Breznitz S (eds): Handbook of Stress: Theoretical and Clinical Aspects. New York, Free Press, 1982

Dunn J: Distress and Comfort. Cambridge, MA, Harvard University Press, 1977

Erickson E: Childhood and Society, 2nd ed. New York, Norton, 1963

Haan N: Coping and Defending: Processes of Self-environment Organization. New York, Academic Press, 1977

Holroyd K, Lazarus R: Stress, coping, and somatic adaption. In Goldberger L, Breynitz S (eds): Handbook of Stress: Theoretical and Clinical Aspects. New York, Free Press, 1982

Janis I: Decision making under stress. In Goldberger L, Breynitz S (eds): Handbook of Stress: Theoretical and Clinical Aspects. New York, Free Press, 1982

Janis I: Stress inoculation in health care. In Meichenbaum D, Jaremko M (eds): Stress Reduction and Prevention. New York, Plenum Press, 1983

Kendall P: Stressful medical procedures. In Meichenbaum D, Jaremko M (eds): Stress Reduction and Prevention. New York, Plenum Press, 1983

Lazarus R: Psychological Stress and the Coping Process. New York, McGraw-Hill, 1966

Lazarus R, Cohen JB, Fokman S, Kanner A, Schaefer C: Psychological stress and adaption: some unresolved issues. In Selye H (ed): Selye's Guide to Stress Research, Vol 1. New York, Van Nostrand Reinhold, 1980

Lazarus R, Launier R: Stress related transactions between persons and environment. In Pervin L, Lewis M (eds): Perspectives in Interactional Psychology. New York, Plenum Press, 1978

Leventhal H, Nerenz D: A model for stress research with some implications for the control of stress disorders. In Meichenbaum D, Jaremko M (eds): Stress Reduction and Prevention. New York, Plenum Press, 1983

McFarland G, Wasli E: Coping-stress-tolerance pattern. In Thompson J, McFarland G, Hirsch S et al: Clinical Nursing. St Louis, CV Mosby, 1986

Meichenbaum D, Cameron R: Stress inoculation training. In Meichenbaum D, Jaremko M (eds): Stress Reduction and Prevention. New York, Plenum Press, 1983

Miller J: Coping with Chronic Illness: Overcoming Powerlessness. Philadelphia, FA Davis, 1982

Moos R, Billings A: Conceptualizing and measuring coping resources and processes. In Goldberger L, Breznitz S (eds): Handbook of Stress: Theoretical and Clinical Aspects. New York, Free Press, 1982

Vaillant GE: Adaptation to Life. Boston, Little, Brown, 1977

Articles

Bandura A: Self-efficacy toward a unifying theory of behavior change. Psychol Rev 84 (2):191–215, 1977

Carnes BA: Concept analysis: dependence. Crit Care Q 6(4):29–39, 1984

Craft M et al: Nursing care in childhood cancer: coping. Am J Nurs 82(3):440–442, 1982

Elliott SM: Denial as an effective mechanism to allay anxiety following a stressful event. J Psychiatr Nurs 18(10):11–15, 1980

Folkman S, Lazarus RS: An analysis of coping in a middle-aged community sample. J Health Soc Behav 21(3)219–239, 1980

Fraser J, Spicka D: Handling the emotional response to disaster. The case for American Red Cross/community mental health collaboration. Ment Health J 17(4):255–264, 1981

Hoover RM, Parnell PK: An inpatient educational group on stress and coping. J Psychosoc Nurs Ment Health Serv 22(6):17–22, 1984

Jack S: When regression becomes a problem. Can Nurs 77(4):31–37, 1981

Jalowiec A, Powers MJ: Stress and coping in hypertensive and emergency room patients. Nurs Res 30(1):10–15, 1981

Korner I: Hope as a method of coping. J Consult Clin Psychol 34(2):134–139, 1970

Lin N, Ensel W, Simeone R, Kuo W: Social support, stressful life events, and illness: a model and empirical test. J Health Soc Behav 20(2):108–119, 1979

McHugh N, Christman N, Johnson J: Preparatory information: what helps and why. Am J Nurs 82(5):780–782, 1982

Murgatroyd S: Coping and the crisis counsellor. Br Guid Counsel 10(2):151–166, 1982

Smith M, Selye H: Reducing the negative effects of stress. Am J Nurs 79(11):1953–1955, 1979

Wollert R, Levy L, Knight B: Help-giving in behavioral control and stress coping self-help groups. Small Gr Behav 13 (2):204–218, 1982

Coping, Ineffective Individual, Related to Maturational or Situational Crisis

Books

Adams J (ed): Understanding and Managing Stress: A Book of Readings. San Diego, University Associates, 1980

Aguilera D, Messick J: Crisis Intervention, Theory and Methodology. St Louis, CV Mosby, 1982

Bullard P: Coping with Stress: A Psychological Survival Manual. Portland, Pro Seminar Press, Inc, 1980

Butler R, Lewis M: Aging and Mental Health. St Louis, CV Mosby, 1977

Caplan G: Principles of Preventive Psychiatry. New York, Basic Books, 1964

Goldberger L, Breznitz S (eds): Handbook of Stress: Theoretical and Clinical Aspects. New York, Free Press, 1982

Greenberg S, Valletutti P: Stress and the Helping Professions. Baltimore, Paul H Brookes Publishers, 1980

Jacobson E: Modern Treatment of Tense Patients. Springfield, IL, Charles C Thomas, 1970

Kutash I, Schlesinger L: Handbook on Stress and Anxiety. San Francisco, Jossey-Bass, 1980

Madders J: Stress and Relaxation. New York, Arco, 1979

McFarland G, Leonard H, Morris M: Nursing Leadership and Management: Contemporary Strategies. New York, John Wiley & Sons, 1984

Meichenbaum D, Jaremko M (eds): Stress Reduction and Prevention. New York, Plenum Press, 1983

Morrice J: Crisis Intervention Studies in Community Care. New York, Pergamon Press, 1976

Parad H: Crisis Intervention: Selected Readings. New York, Family Service Association of America, 1969

Articles

Aguilera D: Stressors in late adulthood. Family Community Health 2:61–69, 1980

Baldwin B: Crisis intervention: an overview of theory and practice. Counseling Psychol 8(2):43–52, 1979

Bandura A: Self-efficacy. Toward a unifying theory of behavior change. Psychol Rev 84:191–215, 1977

Chen M: Applying Yalom's principles to crisis work . . . some intriguing results. J Psychiatr Nurs 16(6):15–22; 27, 1978

Cronin-Stubbs D: Family crisis intervention: a study. J Psychiatr Nurs 16(1):36–44, 1978

Finkelman A: The nurse therapist: outpatient crisis intervention with the chronic psychiatric patient. J Psychiatr Nurs 15(8):27–32, 1977

Fraser J, Spicka D: Handling the emotional response to disaster. Ment Health J 17(4):255–264, 1981

Gaston S: Death and midlife crisis. J Psychiatr Nurs 18(1):31–35, 1980

Goldstein D: Crisis intervention: a brief therapy model. Nurs Clin North Am 13(4):657–663, 1978

Hatch C, Schut L: Description of a crisis-oriented psychiatric home visiting service. J Psychiatr Nurs 18(4):31–35, 1980

Hefferin E: Life-cycle stressors: an overview of research. Fam Community Health 2:71–101, 1980

Jacobson G: Crisis-oriented therapy. Psychiatr Clin North Am 2(1):39–54, 1979

Johnston R: The holistic experience of stress: opportunity for growth or illness. Occup Health Nurs 28:15–18, 1980

Lancaster B, Berkovsky D: An ecological framework for crisis intervention. J Psychiatr Nurs 16(3):17–23, 1978

Little J: Stress during the human life-cycle. Health Visitor 53:373–376, 1980

Phelan L: Crisis intervention: partnership in problem solving. J Psychiatr Nurs 17(9):22–27, 1979

Pritchard M, Proudfoot M: An introduction to stress management: theory and practice. Wash State J Nurs 52:14–18, 1980

Pruett H: Stressors in middle adulthood. Fam Community Health 2:53–60, 1980

Scott D, Oberst M, Dropkin M: A stress-coping model. ANS 3(1):9–23, 1980

Sexsmith D: Stressors in early adulthood. Fam Community Health 2:43–52, 1980

Tillman K, Feinman J: Stress reduction through movement. Point View 18:4–7, 1981

Troxler R, Cook R: Synergy: a technique for managing stress. Crit Care Update 7:34–35; 37, 1980

Wollert R, Levy L, Knight B: Help-giving in behavioral control and stress coping self-help groups. Small Group Behav 13(2):204–218, 1982

Coping, Ineffective Individual, Related to Organic Brain Syndrome

Books

Cameron R, Meichenbaum D: The nature of effective coping and the treatment of stress related problems: a cognitive-behavioral perspective. In Goldberger L,

Breznitz S (eds): Handbook of Stress: Theoretical and Clinical Aspects. New York, Free Press, 1982

Dennis H: Remotivation therapy groups. In Burnside I (ed): Working with the Elderly: Group Process and Techniques. North Scituate, Duxbury Press, 1978

Ebersole P: Establishing reminiscing groups. In Burnside I (ed): Working with the Elderly: Group Process and Techniques. North Scituate, Duxbury Press, 1978

Freedman A, Kaplan H, Sadock B: Modern Synopsis of Comprehensive Textbook of Psychiatry. Baltimore, Williams & Wilkins, 1978

Kim M, McFarland G, McLane A: Classification of Nursing Diagnoses: Proceedings of the Fifth National Conference. St Louis, CV Mosby, 1984

Kim M, McFarland G, McLane A: Pocket Guide to Nursing Diagnoses. St Louis, CV Mosby, 1984

Miller J: Coping with Chronic Illness. Overcoming Powerlessness. Philadelphia, FA Davis, 1982

Moos R, Billings A: Conceptualizing and measuring coping resources and processes. In Goldberger L, Breynitz S (eds): Handbook of Stress: Theoretical and Clinical Aspects. New York, Free Press, 1982

Taulbee L: Reality orientation: a therapeutic group activity for elderly persons. In Burnside I (ed): Working with the Elderly: Group Process and Techniques. North Scituate, Duxbury Press, 1978

Articles

Allen C: Independence through activity: the practice of occupational therapy (psychiatry)—delivering services to psychiatric patients. AJOT 36(11):731–739, 1982

Bartol M: Confusion: recognition and remedy. Reaching the patient. Part 4. Geriatr Nurs 4(4):234–236, 1983

Buckholdt D et al: Therapeutic pretense in reality orientation. Int J Aging Hum Dev 16(3):167–181, 1983

Burnside I: Resource materials. Aids for teaching, learning, and caring for individuals affected by cognitive losses. J Gerontol Nurs 9(2):108–109; 130, 1983

Chenitz W: Confusion: recognition and remedy. The nurse's aide and the confused person. Part 6. Geriatr Nurs 4(4):238–241, 1983

Chivers T, Westwater J: Hospital care of confused elderly people. Nursing (Oxford) 9:393–396, 1980

Feil N: Group work with disoriented nursing home residents. Soc Work With Groups 5(2):57–65, 1982

Hansen L: Treatment of reduced intellectual functioning in alcoholics. J Stud Alcohol 41(1):156–158, 1980

Kiernat J: The use of life review activity with confused nursing home residents. Am J Occup Ther 33(5):306–310, 1979

Lederer A: Confusion: recognition and remedy. Notes on a nursing home. Part 1. Geriatr Nurs 4(4):224–227, 1983

Mackey A: OBS and nursing care. J Gerontol Nurs 9(2):74–79; 83–85, 1983

Mawson D: Organic psychiatric disorders. Extended cognitive state examination. Part 3. Nurs Times 79(25):28–32, 1983

Mezey M: Confusion: recognition and remedy. Implication for the health professions. Part 7. Geriatr Nurs 4(4):241–244, 1983

Richardson K: Confusion: recognition and remedy. Part 5. Geriatr Nurs 4(4):237–238, 1983

Salisbury S et al: Confusion: Recognition and remedy. Separation of the Confused or Integration With the Lucid? Part 3. Geriatr Nurs 4(4):231–233, 1983

Schneider J: The confused patient. Nurs Times 80(4):43–46, 1984
Scott D, Oberst M, Dropkin M: A stress-coping model. ANS 3(1):9–23, 1980
Sidell M: Confused elderly people and community care. Nursing (Oxford) 9:399–402, 1980
Trockman G: Caring for the confused or delirious patient. Am J Nurs 78(9):1495–1499, 1978
Wolanin M: Confusion: recognition and remedy. Scope of the problem and its diagnosis. Part 2. Geriatr Nurs 4(4):227–230, 1983

Depressive Behavior

Books

Beck AT: Depression, Causes and Treatment. Philadelphia, University of Pennsylvania Press, 1972
Burns DD: Feeling Good: The New Mood Therapy. New York, William Morrow, 1980

Articles

Knowles RD: Coping with lethargy. Am J Nurs 81(8):1465, 1981
Knowles RD: Handling depression by identifying anger. Am J Nurs 81(5):968, 1981
Knowles RD: Handling depression through activity. Am J Nurs 81(6):1187, 1981
Knowles RD: Handling depression through positive reinforcement. Am J Nurs 81(7):1353, 1981
Management of the depressed patient: The art and science of compliance. JCP Monograph No. 1, November, 1982. Memphis, TN, Physicians Postgraduate Press, 1982
Mellencamp A: Adolescent depression: a review of the literature, with implications for nursing care. J Psychosoc Nurs Ment Health Serv 19(9):15–20, 1981
Murphy SA: Learned helplessness: from concept to comprehension. Perspect Psychiatr Care 20(1):27–32, 1982

Family Process, Alteration in

Books

Berger M: Beyond the Double bind. New York, Brunner Mazel, 1978
Bowen M: Family Therapy in Clinical Practice. New York, Jason Aronson, 1978
Guerin RJ (ed): Family Therapy, Theory and Practice. New York, Gardner Press, 1976
Gurman A, Kniskern D (eds): Handbook of Family Therapy. New York, Brunner-Mazel, 1981
Haley J: Problem Solving Therapy. San Francisco, Jossey-Bass, 1977
Haley J: Leaving Home. New York, McGraw-Hill, 1980
Kaslow FW (ed): The International Book of Family Therapy. New York, Brunner-Mazel, 1982
Laird J, Allen J: Family theory and practice. In Rosenblatt A, Waldfogel D (eds): Handbook of Clinical Social Work. San Francisco, Jossey-Bass, 1983
Leventhal H, Nerenz D: A model for stress research with some implications for the control of stress disorder. In Meichenbaum D, Jaremko M (eds): Stress Reduction and Prevention. New York, Plenum Press, 1983
Minchin S: Families and Family Theory. Cambridge, MA, Harvard University Press, 1974

Moos R, Billings A: Conceptualizing and measuring coping resources processes. In Goldberger L, Breynitz S (eds): Handbook of Stress Theoretical and Clinical Aspects. New York, Free Press, 1982

Napier Y, Whitaker CA: The Family Crucible. New York, Harper and Row, 1978

Oehrtman SE: Assessment and crisis intervention: a model for the family. In Hall J, Weaver B (eds): Nursing of Families in Crisis. Philadelphia, JB Lippincott, 1974

Palazzoli M et al: Paradox and counterparadox. New York, Jason Araonson, 1978

Reiss O, Oliveri M: Family paradigm and family coping: a proposal for linking the family's intrinsic adaptive capacities to its response to stress. In Kaslow FW (ed): The International Book of Family Therapy. New York, Brunner and Mazel, 1982

Satir V: Conjoint Family Therapy, rev ed. Palo Alto, CA, Science and Behavior Books, 1967

Walkup L: A concept of crisis. In Hall F, Weaver B (eds): Nursing of Families in Crisis. Philadelphia, JB Lippincott, 1974

Watzlawick P, Beavin J, Jackson D: Pragmatics of Human Communication. New York, Norton, 1967

Articles

Auerwald EH: Interdisciplinary versus ecological approach. Fam Proc 7(2):202–215, 1968

Boss P, McCubbin H, Lester G: The corporate exective wife's coping patterns in response to routine husband-father absence. Fam Proc 18(1):79–86, 1979

Goshen-Cottstein E: The mothering of twins, triplets, and quadruplets. Psychiatry 43(9):189–204, 1980

McCubbin H: Integrating coping behavior in family stress theory. J Marriage Fam 41(2):237–244, 1979

Sahu S: Coping with perinatal death. J Reprod Med 26(3):129–132, 1981

Videka-Sherman L: Coping with the death of a child: a study over time. Am J Orthopsychiatr 52(4):688–698, 1982

Fear

Books

Jones P, Jacob D: Anxiety revisited—from a practice perspective. In Kim M, McFarland G, McLane A (eds): Classification of Nursing Diagnoses. St Louis, CV Mosby, 1984

Kaplan H, Freedman A, Sadock B: Comprehensive Textbook of Psychiatry. Baltimore, Williams & Wilkins, 1980

Kim M, McFarland G, McLane A (eds): Pocket Guide to Nursing Diagnoses. St Louis, CV Mosby, 1984

McFarland G, McCann J: Self-perception self-concept pattern. In Thompson J, McFarland G, Hirsch J, et al: Clinical Nursing. St Louis, CV Mosby, 1986

Meldman M, McFarland G, Johnson E: The Problem-Oriented Psychiatric Index and Treatment Plans. St Louis, CV Mosby, 1976

Wilson H, Kneisl C: Psychiatric Nursing. Menlo Park, CA, Addison-Wesley Publishing Co, 1979

Yocom C: The differentiation of fear and anxiety. In Kim M, McFarland G, McLane A (eds): Classification of Nursing Diagnoses. St Louis, CV Mosby, 1984

Grieving, Anticipatory

Books

Aldrich C: Some dynamics of anticipatory grief. In Schoenberg B, Carr A, Peretz D, Kutscher A (eds): Psychological Aspects of Terminal Care. New York, Columbia University Press, 1974

Doyle P: Grief Counseling and Sudden Death. Springfield, IL, Charles C Thomas, 1980

Glaser B, Strauss A: Awareness of Dying. Chicago, Aldine Publishing Co, 1968

Hess P: Loss & grief. In Bower F (ed): Nursing and the Concept of Loss. New York, John Wiley & Sons, 1980

Kim M, McFarland G: Pocket Guide to Nursing Diagnoses. St Louis, CV Mosby, 1984

Kübler-Ross E: On Death and Dying. New York, Macmillan, 1969

Lindemann E: Beyond Grief: Studies in Crisis Intervention. New York, Jason Aronson, 1979

McFarland G, Wasli E: Potential dysfunctional grieving, Dysfunctional grieving. In Kim M, McFarland G, McLane A, (eds): Pocket Guide to Nursing Diagnoses. St Louis, CV Mosby, 1984

Rando T: Module III: concepts of death, dying, grief and loss. In Hospice Education Program for Nurses. (DHHS Pub. No. HRA 81-27). Washington DC, US Government Printing Office, 1981

Articles

Clayton P, Halikas J, Maurice W, Robins E: Anticipatory grief and widowhood. Br J Psychiatry 122, 47–51, 1973

David C: The resurrection-of-the-dead syndrome. Am J Psychother 34(1):119–126, 1980

Dracup K, Breu C: Using nursing research findings to meet the needs of grieving spouses. Nurs Res 27(4):212–216, 1978

Fulton R, Gottesman D: Anticipatory grief: a psychosocial concept reconsidered. Br J Psychiatry 137:45–54, 1980

Fulton R, Gottesman D: Anticipatory grief. Br J Psychiatry 139:79–80, 1981

Friedman S, Chodoff P, Mason J, Hamburg D: Behavioral observations of parents anticipating the death of a child. Pediatrics 32(4):610–625, 1963

Lindemann E: Symptomatology and management of acute grief. Am J Psychiatry 101(2): 141–148, 1944

Parkes C: Anticipatory grief. Br J Psychiatry 138:183, 1981

Pollock G: Mourning and adaptation. Int J Psychoanal 42:341–361, 1961

Stoller E: Effect of experience on nurses' responses to dying and death in the hospital setting. Nurs Res 29(1):35–38, 1980

Grieving, Dysfunctional

Books

Agee J: Grief and the process of aging. In Werner-Beland J (ed): Grief Responses to Long-Term Illness and Disability. Reston, Reston Publishing Co, 1980

Bankoff E: Effects of friendship support on the psychological well-being of widows. In Research in the Interweave of Social Roles: Friendship, Vol 2. JAI Press, 1981

Bowlby J: Loss: Sadness and Depression—Attachment and Loss, Vol III. New York, Basic Books, 1980

Brown M: Maturational losses. In Bower F (ed): Nursing and the Concept of Loss. New York, John Wiley & Sons, 1980

Brown M, Hess P: Nursing and the Concept of Loss. New York, John Wiley & Sons, 1980

Caplan G: Principles of Preventive Psychiatry. New York, Basic Books, 1964

Doyle P: Grief Counseling and Sudden Death. Springfield, IL, Charles C Thomas, 1980

Feifel H: New Meanings of Death. New York, McGraw-Hill, 1977

Glaser B, Strauss A: Awareness of Dying. Chicago, Aldine Publishing Co, 1965

Glaser B, Strauss A: Time for Dying. Chicago, Aldine Publishing Co, 1968

Glick I, Weiss R, Parkes C: The First Year of Bereavement. New York, John Wiley & Sons, 1974

Hess P: Loss and grief. In Bower F (ed): Nursing and the Concept of Loss. New York, John Wiley & Sons, 1980

Jackson E: The pastoral counselor and the child encountering death. In Wass H, Corr C (eds): Helping Children Cope with Death: Guidelines and Resources. New York, Hemisphere Publishing Co, 1982

Kim M, McFarland G, McLane A (eds): Pocket Guide to Nursing Diagnoses. St Louis, CV Mosby, 1984

Kubler-Ross E: On Death and Dying. New York, Macmillan, 1969

Lindemann E: Beyond Grief: Studies in Crisis Intervention. New York, Aronson, 1979

McFarland G, Wasli E: Potential dysfunctional grieving, dysfunctional grieving. In Kim M, McFarland G, McLane A (eds): Pocket Guide to Nursing Diagnoses. St Louis, CV Mosby, 1984

Rando T: Module III: concepts of death, dying, grief and loss. In Hospice Education Program for Nurses (DHHS Pub. No. HRA 81-27). Washington DC, US Government Printing Office, 1981

Simos B: A Time to Grieve. New York, Family Service Association of America, 1979

Simpson M: Dying, Death, and Grief. New York, Plenum Press, 1979

Werner-Beland J, Agee J: Grief Responses to Long-Term Illness and Disability. Reston, Reston Publishing Co, 1980

Articles

Alexy W: Dimensions of psychological counseling that facilitate the grieving process of bereaved parents. J Counsel Psychol 29(5):498–507, 1982

Blanchard C, Blanchard E, Becker J: The young widow: depressive symptomatology throughout the grief process. Psychiatry 39(4):394–399, 1976

Clayton P, Halikas J, Maurice W et al: Anticipatory grief and widowhood. Br J Psychiatry 122(566):47–51, 1973

Constantino R: Bereavement crises intervention for widows in grief and mourning. Nurs Res 30(6):351–353, 1981

David C: The resurrection-of-the-dead syndrome. Am J Psychother 34(1):119–126, 1980

Dimond M: Bereavement and the elderly: a critical review with implications for nursing practice and research. J Adv Nurs 6:461–470, 1981

Dracup K, Breu C: Using nursing research findings to meet the needs of grieving spouses. Nurs Res 27(4):212–216, 1978

Engel G: Grief and grieving. Am J Nurs 64(9):93–98, 1978

Freihofer P, Felton G: Nursing behaviors in bereavement: An exploratory study. Nurs Res 25(5):332–337, 1976

Fulton R, Gottesman D: Anticipatory grief. Br J Psychiatry 139:79–80, 1981

Fulton R, Gottesman D: Anticipatory grief: a psychosocial concept reconsidered. Br J Psychiatry 137:45–54, 1980

Greenblatt M: The grieving spouse. Am J Psychiatry 135(1):43–47, 1978

Hodgkinson P: Treating abnormal grief in the bereaved. Nurs Times 76(3):126–128, 1980

Horowitz M, Wilner N, Marmar C et al: Pathological grief and the activation of latent self-images. Am J Psychiatry 137(10):1157–1162, 1980

Jackson E: Wisely managing our grief: a pastoral viewpoint. Death Educ 3(2):143–155, 1979

Johnson-Soderberg S: Grief themes. ANS 3(4):15–26, 1981

Lamperelli P, Smith J: The grieving process of adoption; an application of principles and techniques. J Psychiatr Nurs 17(10):24–29, 1979

Lindemann E: Symptomatology and management of acute grief. Am J Psychiatry 101:141–148, 1944

McCawley A: Help patients cope with grief. Consultant 17(11):64–67, 1977

Melges F, DeMaso D: Grief-resolution therapy: reliving, revising, and revisiting. Am J Psychother 34(1):51–61, 1980

Parkes C: Anticipatory grief. Br J Psychiatry 138:183, 1981

Pisarcik G: Psychiatric emergencies and crises intervention. Nurs Clin North Am 16(1):85–94, 1981

Raphael B: Preventive intervention with the recently bereaved. Arch Gen Psychiatry 34(12):1450–1454, 1977

Salladay S, Royal M: Children and death: guidelines for grief work. Child Psychiatry Hum Dev 11(4):203–212, 1981

Schmale A: Reactions to illness; convalescence and grieving. Psychiatr Clin North Am 2(2):321–330, 1979

Schultz C: The dynamics of grief. J Emerg Nurs 5(5):26–30, 1979

Sease S: Grief associated with a prison experience: Counseling the client. J Psychiatr Nurs Men Health Serv 20(7):25–27, 1982

Stoller E: Effect of experience on nurses' responses to dying and death in the hospital setting. Nurs Res 29(1):35–38, 1980

Thomas G: Human grief when a pet dies, Part 1. Cincinnati Horiz 12(4):8–11, 1983

Vachon M: Grief and bereavement following the death of a spouse. Can Psychiatr Assoc J 21(1):35–43, 1976

Weingourt R: Battered women: the grieving process. J Psychiatr Nurs 17(4):40–47, 1979

Wilson A, Fenton L, Stevens D, Soule D: The death of a newborn twin: an analysis of parental bereavement. Pediatrics 70(4):587–591, 1982

Wylie N, Kustaborder M: Helping caregivers cope with loss, especially dying. J Gerontol Nurs 7(8):469–473, 1981

Guilt

Book

Beck CM, Rawlins RP, Williams SR: Mental Health Psychiatric Nursing: A Holistic Life-Cycle Approach. St Louis, CV Mosby, 1984

Articles

Knowles RD: Managing guilt. Am J Nurs 81(10):1850, 1981

Knowles RD: Overcoming guilt and worry. Am J Nurs 81(9):1663, 1981

Knowles RD: Worry journal and guilty time. Am J Nurs 81(11):20–35, 1981

Hyperactive Behavior

Article

Loney J: Hyperkinesis comes of age: What do we know and where should we go? Am J Orthopsychiatry 50(1):28–42, 1980

Knowledge Deficit (Specify)

Books

Bille DA (ed): Practical Approaches to Patient Teaching. Boston, Little, Brown, 1981

Bloom BS (ed): Taxonomy of Educational Objectives: The Classification of Educational Goals. Handbook I. Cognitive Domain. New York, McKay, 1956

Chatham MAH, Knapp BL: Patient Education Handbook. Bowie, MD, Brady, 1982

Doak CCD, Doak LG, Root JH: Teaching Patients with Low Literacy Skills. Philadelphia, Lippincott, 1985

Gagne RM: Principles of Instructional Design, 2nd ed. New York, Holt, Rinehart and Winston, 1979

Harrow AJ: A taxonomy of the Psychomotor Domain. New York, McKay, 1972

Joyce B, Weil M: Models of Teaching. Englewood Cliffs, NJ, Prentice-Hall, 1980

Kibler RJ et al: Objectives for Instruction and Evaluation, 2nd ed. Boston, Allyn & Bacon, 1981

Krathwohl DR, Bloom BS, Masia BB: Taxonomy of Educational Objectives: The Classification of Educational Goals. Handbook II. Affective Domain. New York, McKay, 1964

Megenity JS, Megenity J: Patient Teaching: Theories, Techniques and Strategies. Bowie, MD, Brady, 1982

Rankin SL, Duffy KL: Patient Education: Issues, Principles, and Guidelines. Philadelphia, JB Lippincott, 1983

Redman BK (ed): Issues and Concepts in Patient Education. New York, Appleton-Century-Crofts, 1981

Redman BK: The Process of Patient Education, 5th ed. St Louis, CV Mosby, 1984

Squyres WD (ed): Patient Education: An Inquiry into the State of the Art. New York, Springer-Verlag, 1980

Articles

Becker MH. The health belief model and sick role behavior. Health Educ Monogr 2:409–419, 1974

Manic Behavior

Articles

Bjork D, Steinberg M, Lindenmayer J, Pardes H: Mania and milieu; treatment of manics in a therapeutic community. Hosp Community Psychiatry 28(6):431–436, 1977

Hussey T: Manic-depressive psychosis with rapid and profound changes of mood. Nurs Times 75(5):193–195, 1979

Janowsky DS, Leff M, Epstein RS: Playing the manic game: interpersonal maneuvers of the acutely manic patient. Arch Gen Psychiatry 22(3):252–261, 1970

Manipulation

Books

Bursten B: The Manipulator: The Psychoanalytic View. New Haven, Yale University Press, 1973

Meldman M, McFarland G, Johnson E: The problem-oriented psychiatric index and treatment plan. St Louis, CV Mosby, 1976

Articles

Carser D: The defense mechanism of splitting: developmental origins, effects on staff, recommendations for nursing care. J Psychiatr Nurs 17(3):21–28, 1979

McMorrow ME: The manipulative patient. Am J Nurs 81(6):188–190, 1981

Noncompliance

Articles

Amarasingham LR: Social and cultural perspectives on medication refusal. Am J Psychiatry 137(3):353–358, 1980

Connelly CE: Patient compliance: a review of the research with implications for psychiatric-mental health nursing. J Psychiatr Nurs 16(10):15–18, 1978

del Campo JH, Carr CF, Correa E: Rehospitalized schizophrenics: what they report about illness, treatment, and compliance. J Psychosoc Nurs Ment Health Serv 21(6):29–33, 1983

Jamison KR, Akiskal HS: Medication compliance in patients with bipolar disorder. Psychiatr Clin North Am 6(1):175–192, 1983

McMorrow MJ, Cullinan D, Epstein MH: The use of the premack principle to motivate patient activity attendance. Perspect Psychiatr Care 16(1): 14–18, 1978

Todd B: 27 reasons people don't take their meds. RN 44(3):54–57, 1981

Physical Symptoms, Inappropriate Use of

Article

Hall RC, Gardner ER, Stickney SK et al: Physical illness manifesting as psychiatric disease. Arch Gen Psychiatry 37(9):989–995, 1980

Powerlessness

Books

Blau P: Exchange and Power in Social Life. New York, John Wiley & Sons, 1964

French J, Raven B: The bases of social power. In Cartwright D (ed): Studies in Social Power. Ann Arbor, The University of Michigan, 1959

Kim M, McFarland G, McLane A (eds): Pocket Guide to Nursing Diagnoses. St Louis, CV Mosby, 1984

McFarland G, Leonard H, Morris M: Nursing Leadership and Management: Contemporary Strategies. New York, John Wiley & Sons, 1984

Meldman M, McFarland G, Johnson E: The Problem Oriented Psychiatric Index and Treatment Plans. St Louis, CV Mosby, 1976

Miller J: Coping With Chronic Illness: Overcoming Powerlessness. Philadelphia, FA Davis, 1983

Mills W: Alienation: A basic concept underlying social isolation. In Kim M, McFarland G, McLane A (eds): Classification of Nursing Diagnoses: Proceedings of the Fifth National Conference. St Louis, CV Mosby, 1984

Seligman M: Helplessness: On Depression, Development, and Death. San Francisco, WH Freeman, 1975

Thompson J, McFarland G, Hirsch J et al: Clinical Nursing. St Louis, CV Mosby, 1986

Articles

Adelson P: The backward dilemma. Am J Nurs 80(3):423–425, 1980

Arakelian M: An assessment and nursing application of the concept of locus of control. ANS 3(1):25–42, 1980

Bachrach L: A conceptual approach to deinstitutionalization. Hosp Community Psychiatry 29(9):573–578, 1978

Craig A, Hyatt B: Chronicity in mental illness: a theory on the role of change. Perspect Psychiatr Care 16(3):139–154, 1978

Glass C, Levy L: Perceived psychophysiological control: the effects of power versus powerlessness. Cog Ther Res 6(1):91–103, 1982

Jenkins L: The concept of assertion: from theory to practice. Issues Ment Health Nurs 4:51–63, 1982

Rotter J: Generalized expectancies for internal versus external control of reinforcement. Psychol Monogr Gen Appl (Whole No. 609) 80(1):1–28, 1966

Schmidt M: Exchange and power in special settings for the aged. Int J Aging Hum Dev 14(3):157–166, 1981–1982

Slavinsky A, Krauss J: Mutual withdrawal . . . or Gwen Tudor revisited. Perspect Psychiatr Care 18(5):194–203, 1980

Weinberg J: The chronic patient: the stranger in our midst. Hosp Community Psychiatry 29(1):25–28, 1978

Ritualistic Behavior

Article

Hagerty BK: Obsessive-compulsive behavior: an overview of four psychological frameworks. J Psychosoc Nurs Ment Health Serv 19(1):37–39, 1981

Self-Care Deficit

Article

Jack S: When regression becomes a problem. Can Nurs 77(4):31–37, 1981

Self-Concept, Disturbance in: Body Image

Books

Bonham P, Cheney A: Concept of self: a framework for nursing assessment. In Chinn P (ed): Advances in Nursing Theory Development. Rockville, MD, Aspen Systems, 1983

Combs A, Snygg D: Individual Behavior: a Perceptual Approach to Behavior. New York, Harper & Row, 1959

Fitts W: The Self-concept and Self-actualization. Nashville, Dede Wallace Center, 1971

Kim M, McFarland G, McLane A (eds): Classification of Nursing Diagnoses; Proceedings of the Fifth National Conference. St Louis, CV Mosby, 1984

Kim M, McFarland G, McLane A: Pocket Guide to Nursing Diagnoses. St Louis, CV Mosby, 1984

McFarland G, McCann J: Self-perception self-concept pattern. In Thompson J, McFarland G, Hirsch J et al: Clinical Nursing. St Louis, CV Mosby, 1986

Articles

McCloskey J: How to make the most of body image theory in nursing practice. Nursing '76 6(5):68-72, 1976

Murray R (ed): The concept of body image. Nurs Clin North Am 7(4):593-707, 1972

Self-Concept, Disturbance in: Self-Esteem

Books

Bonham P, Cheney A: Concept of self: a framework for nursing assessment. In Chinn P (ed): Advances in Nursing Theory Development. Rockville, MD, Aspen Systems, 1983

Clark C: Assertive Skills for Nurses. Wakefield, Contemporary Publishing, 1978

Fitts W: The Self Concept and Performance. Nashville, Dede Wallace Center, 1972

Fitts W: The Self Concept and Psychopathology. Nashville, Dede Wallace Center, 1972

Hamachek D: Encounters with the Self. New York, Holt, Rinehart, & Winston, 1971

Kim M, McFarland G, McLane A: Pocket Guide to Nursing Diagnoses. St Louis, CV Mosby, 1984

Lewis G: Nurse-Patient Communication. Dubuque, Wm C Brown Co., 1978

McFarland G, McCann J: Self-concept-self-perception pattern. In Thompson J, McFarland G, Hirsch J et al: Clinical Nursing. St Louis, CV Mosby, 1986

Meldman M, McFarland G, Johnson E: The Problem-Oriented Psychiatric Index and Treatment Plans. St Louis, CV Mosby, 1976

Moskowitz R: Assertiveness for Career and Personal Success. New York, American Management Association, 1977

Rosenberg M: Conceiving the Self. New York, Basic Books, 1979

Taylor M: The need for self-esteem. In Yura H, Walsh M (eds): Human Needs and the Nursing Process. Norwalk, CT, Appleton-Century-Crofts, 1982

Articles

Andreoli K: Self-concept and health beliefs in compliant and non-compliant hypertensive patients. Nurs Res 30:323-328, 1981

Antonucci T et al: Physical health and self-esteem. Fam Community Health 6(2):1-9, 1983

Callis C: Appearance programs with female chronic psychiatric hospital patients: a comparison of six-week and nine-week treatment interventions—one's clothing may be operant in restoring feelings of self-worth. J Rehabil 48(4):34-39, 1982

Crouch M: Future needs for self-esteem research and services. Fam Community Health 6(2):70-81, 1983

Crouch M et al: Enhancement of self-esteem in adults. Fam Community Health 6(2):65-78, 1983

Gilberts R: The evaluation of self-esteem. Fam Community Health 6(2):29-49, 1983

Hirst S et al: Promoting self-esteem. J Gerontol Nurs 10(2):72-77, 1984

Goldberg C, Stanitis M: The enhancement of self-esteem through the communication process in group therapy. J Psychiatr Nurs 15(12):5-8, 1977

Knowles R: Dealing with feelings: control your thoughts. Am J Nurs 81(2):353, 1981

Reasoner R: Enhancement of self-esteem in children and adolescents. Fam Community Health 6(2):51–64, 1983

Riffee D: Self-esteem changes in hospitalized school-age children. Nurs Res 30(2):94–97, 1981

Stanwyck D: Self-esteem through the life span. Fam Community Health 6(2):11–28, 1983

Tinelli S: The relationship of family concept to individual self-esteem. Issues Ment Health Nurs 3:251–270, 1981

Sensory/Perceptual Alteration

Articles

Field WE, Ruelke W: Hallucinations and how to deal with them. Am J Nurs 73(4):638–640, 1973

Schwartzman ST: The hallucinating patient and nursing intervention. J Psychiatr Nurs 13(6):23–36, 1975

Sexual Dysfunction

Articles

Akhtar S, Crocker E, Dickey N et al: Overt sexual behavior among psychiatric inpatients. Dis Nerv Syst 38(5):359–361, 1977

Assey JL, Herbert JM: Who is the seductive patient? Am J Nurs 83(4):530–532, 1983

Elmassian BJ, Wilson RN: Assessment and diagnosis of sexual problems. Nurs Pract 7(6):13–22, 1982

Hampton PJ: Coping with the male patient's sexuality. Nurs Forum 18(3):304–310, 1979

Paradowski W: Socialization patterns and sexual problems of the institutionalized chronically ill and physically disabled. Arch Phys Med Rehabil 58(2):53–59, 1977

Shaul S, Morrey L: Sexuality education in a state mental hospital. Hosp Community Psychiatry 31(3):175–179, 1980

Social Isolation

Books

Curran JP, Monti PM (eds): Social Skills Training: A Practical Handbook for Assessment and Treatment. New York, Guilford Press, 1982

Mills WC: Alienation: A basic concept underlying social isolation. In Kim MJ, McFarland GK, McLane AM (eds): Classification of Nursing Diagnosis: Proceedings of the Fifth National Conference. St Louis, CV Mosby, 1984

Articles

Brady JP: Social skills training for psychiatric patients, I: Concepts, methods, and clinical results. Am J Psychiatry 141(3):333–340, 1984

Marlowe HA, Marcotte A: Client skills: non-verbal decoding. J Psychosoc Nurs 22(4):8–15, 1984

Schmidt CS: Withdrawal behavior of schizophrenics: application of Roy's model. J Psychosoc Nurs Ment Health Serv 19(11):26–33, 1981

Tudor G: A sociopsychiatric nursing approach to intervention in a problem of mutual withdrawal on a mental hospital ward. Perspect Psychiatr Care 8(1):11–35, 1970

Spiritual Distress

Books

Colliton M: The spiritual dimensions of nursing. In Beland I, Passos J. Clinical Nursing: Pathophysiological and Psychosocial Approaches. New York, Macmillan, 1981

Fish S, Shelly J: Spiritual Care: The Nurse's Role. Downers Grove, Inter-Varsity Press, 1978

Henderson V, Nite G: Principles and Practice of Nursing. New York, Macmillan, 1978

Kim M, McFarland G, McLane A (eds): Classification of Nursing Diagnoses: Proceedings of the Fifth National Conference. St Louis, CV Mosby, 1984

Kim M, McFarland G, McLane A (eds): Pocket Guide to Nursing Diagnoses. St Louis, CV Mosby, 1984

Moberg D: The development of social indicators of spiritual well-being for quality of life research. In Moberg D (ed): Spiritual Well-Being: Sociological Perspectives. Washington DC, University Press of America, 1979

O'Brien M: The need for spiritual integrity. In Yura H, Walsh M (eds): Human Needs and the Nursing Process. Norwalk, CT, Appleton-Century-Crofts, 1982

Paloritzian R, Ellison C: Loneliness, spiritual well-being, and quality of life. In Peplau L, Perlman D: Loneliness: A Sourcebook of Current Theory, Research, and Therapy. New York, John Wiley & Sons, 1983

Spiritual Perspectives, Vols. I & II (Reprints from The Nurses Lamp). Madison, WI Nurses Christian Fellowship, 1969–1978

Stallwood J, Stoll R: Spiritual dimensions of nursing practice. In Beland I, Passos J (eds): Clinical Nursing: Pathophysiological and Psychosocial Approaches. New York, Macmillan, 1975

Articles

Buys A: Discussion series sensitizes nurses to patients' spiritual needs. Hosp Progress 62:44, 1981

Carson V: Meeting the spiritual needs of hospitalized psychiatric patients. Perspect Psychiatr Care 18(1):17–20, 1980

Carson V, Huss K: Prayer—an effective therapeutic and teaching tool. J. Psychiatr Nurs 17(3):34–37, 1979

Dickinson C: The search for spiritual meaning. Am J Nurs 75(10):1789–1793, 1975

Ellis D: Whatever happened to spiritual dimension? Can Nurse 76:42, 1980

Gilloway F, Donnelly L: Religion and patient care: the functionalist approach. J Adv Nurs 2(1):3–13, 1977

Highfield M, Cason C: Spiritual needs of patients: Are they recognized? Cancer Nurs 6(3):187–192, 1983

O'Brien M: Religious faith and adjustment to long-term hemodialysis. J Relig Health 21:68, 1982

Piepgras R: The other dimension: spiritual help. Am J Nurs 68(12):2610–2613, 1968

Pumphrey J: Recognizing your patients' spiritual needs. Nursing '77 7(12):64–70, 1977

Stoll R: Guidelines for spiritual assessment. Am J Nurs 79(9):1574–1577, 1979

Substance Abuse (Alcohol)

Books

Barnard C: Families, Alcoholism, and Therapy. Springfield, IL, Charles C Thomas, 1981

Bean M, Zinberg N (eds): Dynamic Approaches to the Understanding and Treatment of Alcoholism: The Nature of Alcoholism and the Care of the Alcoholic. New York, Free Press, 1981

Diagnostic and Statistical Manual of Mental Disorders, DSM-III. Washington DC, American Psychiatric Association, 1982

Edwards G, Grant M (eds): Alcoholism Treatment in Transition. Baltimore, University Park Press, 1980

Estes N, Heinemann M: Alcoholism: Development, Consequences, and Interventions. St Louis, CV Mosby, 1977

Ewing J, Rouse B: Drinking, Alcohol in American Society—Issues and Current Research. Chicago, Nelson-Hall, 1978

Fann W et al (eds): Phenomenology and Treatment of Alcoholism: Symposium on Phenomenology and Treatment of Alcoholism. New York, SP Medical & Scientific Books, 1980

Forrest G: Alcoholism, Narcissism, and Psychopathology. Springfield, IL, Charles C Thomas, 1983

Gitlow S, Peyser H (eds): Alcoholism: A Practical Treatment Guide. New York, Grune & Stratton, 1980

Glaser F, Greenberg S, Barrett M: A Systems Approach to Alcohol Treatment. Toronto, Addiction Research Foundation, 1978

Goby M (ed): Alcoholism: A New Frontier for Health Care Institutions. St Louis, Catholic Health Association of the United States, 1983

Gottheil E et al (eds): Alcohol, Drug Abuse, and Aggression. Springfield, IL, Charles C Thomas, 1983

Gottheil E et al (eds): The Combined Problems of Alcoholism, Drug Addiction, and Aging. Springfield, IL, Charles C Thomas, 1984

Gottheil E, McLellan A, Druley K (eds): Substance Abuse and Psychiatric Illness: Proceedings of the Second Annual Coatesville-Jefferson Conference on Addiction. New York, Pergamon Press, 1980

Gottheil E, McLellan A, Druley K (eds): Matching Patient Needs and Treatment Methods in Alcoholism and Drug Abuse. Springfield, IL, Charles C Thomas, 1981

Hay W, Nathan P (eds): Clinical Case Studies in the Behavioral Treatment of Alcoholism. New York, Plenum Press, 1982

Kaufman E (ed): The Power to Change: Family Case Studies in the Treatment of Alcoholism. New York, Gardner Press, 1983

Lawson G, Peterson J, Lawson A: Alcoholism and the Family: A Guide to Treatment and Prevention. Rockville, Aspen Systems, 1983

Madden J: A Guide to Alcohol and Drug Dependence. Bristol, John Wright & Sons, 1979

McEwan R: Education for the Nursing Role in Alcoholism Treatment. Wellington, Alcoholic Liquor Advisory Council, 1981

Murray R, Huelskoetter M: Psychiatric Mental Health Nursing: Giving Emotional Care. Englewood Cliffs, NJ, Prentice-Hall, 1983

Powell D (ed): Alcoholism and Sexual Dysfunction. New York, Haworth Press, 1984

Solomon J (ed): Alcoholism and Clinical Psychiatry. New York, Plenum Medical Books, 1982

Solomon S: Tailoring Alcoholism Therapy to Client Needs (ADM) 81-1129. Rockville, MD, US Department of Health and Human Services, 1981

Volpe J: Advances in Alcoholism Treatment Services for Women (ADM)83-1217. Rockville, MD, US Department of Health and Human Services, 1983

Ward D (ed): Alcoholism: Introduction to Theory and Treatment. Dubuque, Kendall/Hunt, 1980

Zimberg S: The Clinical Management of Alcoholism. New York, Brunner/Mazel, 1982

Articles

Berger F: Alcoholism rehabilitation: a supportive approach. Hosp Comm Psychiatry 34(11):1040–1043, 1983

Brown L, Ostrow F: The development of an assertiveness program on an alcoholism unit. Int J Addict 15(3):323–327, 1980

Caddy G, Addington H, Perkins D: Individualized behavior therapy for alcoholics: a third year independent double-blind follow-up. Behav Res Ther 16(5):345–362, 1978

Crook T, Cohen G: Future directions for research on alcohol and the elderly. Alcohol Health Res World 8(3):25–29, 1984

Crovella A: When your patient's an alcoholic. RN 47(2):50–53, 1984

Crumbaugh J, Carr G: Treatment of alcoholics with logotherapy. Int J Addict 14(6):847–853, 1979

Finlay D: Alcoholism and systems theory: building a better mousetrap. Psychiatry 41(3):272–278, 1978

Fischer J: The relationship between alcoholic patients' milieu perception and measures of their drinking during a brief follow-up period. Int J Addict 14(8):1151–1156, 1979

Freund G: Current research directions on alcohol problems and aging. Alcohol Health Res World 8(3):11–15, 1984

Gareri E: Assertiveness training for alcoholics. J Psychiatr Nurs 17(1):31–36, 1979

Gilbert G, Parker J, Claiborn C: Differential mood changes in alcoholics as a function of anxiety management strategies. J Clin Psychol 34(1):229–232, 1978

Goodwin D: The genetics of alcoholism. Hosp Comm Psychiatry 34(11):1031–1034, 1983

Halikas J: Psychotropic medication used in the treatment of alcoholism. Hosp Comm Psychiatry 34(11):1035–1039, 1983

Hinrichsen J: Toward improving treatment services for alcoholics of advanced age. Alcohol Health Res World 8(3):31–39, 1984

Hirsch S, Rosenberg R, Phelan C et al: Effectiveness of assertiveness training with alcoholics. J Stud Alcohol 39(1):89–97, 1978

Hogen J: Alcoholism treatment: an unfilled prescription. RN 47(1):71, 1984

Intagliata J: Increasing the interpersonal problem-solving skills of an alcoholic population. J Consult Clin Psychol 46(3):489–498, 1978

Kennedy R, Gilbert G, Thoreson R: A self-control program for drinking antecedents: the role of self-monitoring and control orientation. J Clin Psychol 34(1):238–243, 1978

Kurtines W, Ball L, Wood C: Personality characteristics of long-term recovered alcoholics: a comparative analysis. J Consult Clin Psychol 46(5):971–977, 1978

MacDonough T: Evaluation of the effectiveness of intensive confrontation in changing the behavior of alcohol and drug abusers. Int J Addict 13(4):529–589, 1978

McCourt W, Glantz M: Cognitive behavior therapy in groups for alcoholics. J Stud Alcohol 41(3):338–346, 1980

McFarland G, Apostoles F: The nursing history in a psychiatric setting: adaptation to a variety of nursing care patterns and patient populations. J Psychiatr Nurs 13(4):12–17, 1975

Miller W: Behavior treatment of problem drinkers: a comparative outcome study of three controlled drinking therapies. J Consult Clin Psychol 46(1):74–86, 1978

Moos R, Bromet E: Relation of patient attributes to perceptions of the treatment environment. J Consult Clin Psychol 46(2):350–351, 1978

Owen P: A multimodal treatment approach for incarcerated alcoholics. J Clin Psychol 34(4):1005–1009, 1978

Page R, Schaub L: EMG biofeedback applicability for differing personality types. J Clin Psychol 34(4):1014–1020, 1978

Pallikkathayil L, Tweed S: Substance abuse: alcohol and drugs during adolescence. Nurs Clin North Am 18(2):313–321, 1983

Parker J, Gilbert G: Reduction of autonomic arousal in alcoholics: a comparison of relaxation and meditation techniques. J Consult Clin Psychol 46(5):879–886, 1978

Schuckit M: Alcoholism and other psychiatric disorders. Hosp Comm Psychiatry 34(11):1022–1027, 1983

Segal M et al: The 1990 prevention objectives for alcohol and drug misuse: progress report. Public Health Rep 98(5):426–435, 1983

Smith J: Diagnosing alcoholism. Hosp Comm Psychiatry 34(11):1017–1021, 1983

Thompson M et al: Alcohol education in schools: toward a lifestyle risk-reduction approach. J Sch Health 54(2):79–82, 1984

Twerski A: Early intervention in alcoholism: confrontational techniques. Hosp Comm Psychiatry 34(11):1027–1030, 1983

Van Gee S: Alcoholism and the family: a psychodrama appraoch. J Psychiatr Nurs 17(8):9–12, 1979

Vannicelli M: Treatment contracts in an inpatient alcoholism treatment setting. J Stud Alcohol 40(5):457–471, 1979

Substance Abuse (Drugs)

Books

Assessing Treatment: The Conduct of Evaluation within Drug Abuse Treatment Programs (ADM)82-1218. Rockville, MD, US Department of Health and Human Services, 1982

Baron J: Kids and Drugs: A Parent's Handbook of Drug Abuse Prevention and Treatment. New York, Perigee Books, 1984

Bennett J, Demos G: Drug Abuse and What We Can Do About It. Springfield, IL, Charles C Thomas, 1972

Brill L: The Clinical Treatment of Substance Abusers. New York, Free Press, 1981

Craig R, Baker S: Drug Dependent Patients: Treatment and Research. Springfield, IL, Charles C Thomas, 1982

Davis C, Schmidt M: Differential Treatment of Drug and Alcohol Abusers. Palm Springs, FL, ETC Publications, 1977

Drug Use and Misuse: A Growing Concern for Older Americans. Washington DC, US Government Printing Office, 1983

European Public Health Committee: Treatment of Drug Dependence: Final Report. Strasbourg, Council of Europe, 1980

Gardner S (ed): Drug and Alcohol Abuse: Implications for Treatment (ADM)

80-958. Rockville, MD, US Department of Health and Human Services, 1981

Gottheil E et al: Alcohol, Drug Abuse, and Aggression. Springfield, IL, Charles C Thomas, 1983

Gottheil E et al: The Combined Problems of Alcoholism, Drug Addiction, and Aging. Springfield, IL, Charles C Thomas, 1984

Gottheil E, McLellan A, Druley K (eds): Substance Abuse and Psychiatric Illness: Proceedings of the Second Annual Coatesville-Jefferson Conference on Addiction. New York, Pergamon Press, 1980

Gottheil E, McLellan A, Druley K (eds): Matching Patient Needs and Treatment Methods in Alcoholism and Drug Abuse. Springfield, IL, Charles C Thomas, 1981

Senay E et al: The Primary Physician's Guide to Drug Abuse Treatment (ADM)82-1194. Rockville, MD, US Department of Health and Human Services, 1982

Senay E, Becker C, Schnoll S, Dendy R (eds): Emergency Treatment of the Drug Abusing Patient (ADM)80-1023. Rockville, MD, US Department of Health and Human Services, 1980

Smart R: Forbidden Highs: The Nature, Treatment, and Prevention of Illicit Drug Abuse. Toronto, Addiction Research Foundation, 1983

Sobell L, Sobell M, Ward E (eds): Evaluating Alcohol and Drug Abuse Treatment Effectiveness: Recent Advances. New York, Pergamon Press, 1980

Wilford B: Drug Abuse: A Guide for the Primary Care Physician. Chicago, American Medical Association, 1981

Articles

Abruzzi W: The failure of therapeutic communities, drug treatment, and rehabilitation programs. Int J Addict 14(7):1023-1030, 1979

Andersen M: Personalized nursing: a unique approach to drug-dependent women. JEN 8(5):225-231, 1982

Coleman S, Davis D: Family therapy and drug abuse: a national survey. Fam Process 17(1):21-29, 1978

Collins J et al: Legal coercion and retention in drug abuse treatment. J Hosp Comm Psychiatry 34(12):1145-1149, 1983

Dietch J: The nature and extent of benzodiazepine abuse: an overview of recent literature. Hosp Comm Psychiatry 34(12):1139-1145, 1983

Doyle K et al: Treating the drug abuser. Public Health Rev 10(1):77-98, 1982

Family therapy helps addict: JAMA 241(6):546-551, 1979

Gossop M: Drug dependence—1. The pattern of drug abuse. Nurs Times 74(23):996-998, 1978

Gossop M: Drug dependence—2. Treatment and nursing care. Nurs Times 74(25):1060-1061, 1978

Hodgman C: Current issues in adolescent psychiatry. Hosp Comm Psychiatry 34(6):514-521, 1983

Huberty D, Malmquist J: Adolescent chemical dependency. Perspect Psychiatr Care 16(1):21-27, 1978

Johnson E, Klotkowski D: Turning an addicted patient on to turning drugs off. RN 41(5):91-97, 1978

Kittleson M et al: Primary prevention and implications for drug education programs. Health Values 6(6):30-35, 1982

Klagsbrun M, Davis D: Substance abuse and family interaction. Fam Process 16(2):149-173, 1977

O'Brien J: Behavioral problems due to substance abuse. Top Emerg Med 4(4):30–41, 1983

Pallikkathayil L, Tweed S: Substance abuse: alcohol and drugs during adolescence. Nurs Clin North Am 18(2):313–321, 1983

Panyard C, Wolf K: Attitudinal differences affecting participation in group counseling in outpatient drug treatment centers. Int J Addict 14(7):987–992, 1979

Personett J: Couples therapy: treatment of choice with the drug addict. J Psychiatr Nurs 16(1):18–21, 1978

Quinones M, Doyle K, Sheffet A et al: Evaluation of drug abuse rehabilitation efforts: a review. Am J Public Health 69(11):1164–1169, 1979

Rice M et al: Review: identifying the adolescent substance abuser. MCN 8(2):139–142, 1983

Segal M et al: The 1990 prevention objectives for alcohol and drug misuse: progress report. Public Health Rep 98(5):426–435, 1983

Shestowsky B: Health care needs of residents in an alcohol and drug rehabilitation centre. Can J Psychiatr Nurs 24(3):12, 1983

Smith T: The dynamics in time-limited relationship therapy with methadone-maintained patients. Perspect Psychiatr Care 16(1):28–33, 1978

Stanton M: Family treatment approaches to drug abuse problems: a review. Fam Process 18(3):251–275, 1979

Stanton M: The addict as savior: heroin, death, and the family. Fam Process 16(2):191–197, 1977

Todd B: Addicted or physically dependent? Geriatr Nurs 5(1):59; 62, 1984

Toohey J et al: Rehabilitating the school age drug abuser in an institutional setting. Health Educ 13(6):50–52, 1982

Weller R, Halikas J: Objective criteria for the diagnosis of marijuana abuse. J Nerv Ment Dis 168(2):98–103, 1980

Suicide, Potential

Books

Clarkin J, Glazer H (eds): Depression, Behavioral and Directive Intervention Strategies. New York, Garland STPM Press, 1981

Clinical Center Nursing Department. Suicide Prevention: The Challenge for Nurses. NIH Publication No. 82-2308. Bethesda, MD, Department of Health and Human Services, 1981

Gallagher D, Thompson L: Depression in the Elderly. Los Angeles, Andrus Gerontology Center, 1981

Hawton K, Catalian J: Attempted Suicide, A Practical Guide to Its Nature and Management. Oxford, Oxford University Press, 1982

Kiev A: The Suicidal Patient: Recognition and Management. Chicago, Nelson-Hall, 1977

Kiev A: The prevention of suicide. In Masserman J (ed): Current Psychiatric Therapies, Vol 18, pp 91–95. New York, Grune & Stratton, 1979

McIntire M, Angle C (eds): Suicide Attempts in Children and Youth. Hagerstown, MD, Harper & Row, 1980

Miller M: Suicide Prevention by Nurses. New York, Springer-Verlag, 1982

Rehm L (ed): Behavior Therapy for Depression: Present Status and Future Directions. New York, Academic Press, 1981

Reynolds D, Farberow N: The Family Shadow: Sources of Suicide and Schizophrenia. Berkeley, University of California Press, 1981

Wells C, Stuart I (eds): Self Destructive Behavior in Children and Adolescents. New York, Van Nostrand Reinhold, 1981

Articles

Bascue L et al: Recognition of suicidal lethality factors by psychiatric nursing assistants. Psychol Rep 51(1):197–198, 1982

Beck A, Kovacs M: Assessment of suicidal intention: the scale for suicide ideation. J Consult Clin Psychol 47(2):343–352, 1979

Bressler B: Depression and suicide. Consultant 18(3):123–126; 129, 1978

Busteed E et al: The development of suicide precautions for an inpatient psychiatric unit. J Psychosoc Nurs Ment Health Serv 21(5):15–19, 1983

Capodanno A et al: Assessment of suicide risk: some limitations in the prediction of infrequent events. J Psychosoc Nurs Ment Health Serv 21(5):11–14, 1983

Cotton P et al: Dealing with suicide on a psychiatric inpatient unit. Hosp Comm Psychiatry 34(1):55–59, 1983

DiVasto P, West D, Christy J: A framework for the emergency evaluation of the suicidal patient. J Psychiatr Nurs 17(6):15–20, 1979

Eggland E: Dealing with tragedy: the aftermath of suicide. J Nurs Care 11(12):14–15, 1978

Feinsilver D: The suicidal patient: clinical and legal issues. Hosp Pract 18(10):48E–F; 48J; 48L; 1983

Fitzpatrick J: Suicidology and suicide prevention: historical perspectives from the nursing literature. J Psychosoc Nurs Ment Health Serv 21(5):20–28, 1983

Frances A et al: A suicide attempt by a seductive patient: what's the treatment plan? Hosp Community Psychiatry 33(12):977–979, 1982

Gilead M et al: Adolescent suicide: a response to developmental crisis. Perspect Psychiatr Care 21(3):94–101, 1983

Glinsky J: Stop! Look! Listen! . . . first open suicidal thoughts. Can J Psychiatr Nurse 23(4):11–12, 1982

Gurrister L, Kane R: How therapists perceive and treat suicidal patients. Community Ment Health J 14(1):3–13, 1978

Hafen B et al: Preventing adolescent suicide. Nursing 83 13(10):46–48, 1983

Hopper K, Guttmacher S: Re-thinking suicide notes toward a critical epidemiology. Int J Health Serv 9(3):417–438, 1979

Keidel G: Adolescent suicide. Nurs Clin North Am 18(2):323–332, 1983

Neimeyer R: Toward a personal construct conceptualization of depression and suicide. Death Educ 7(2–3):127–173, 1983

Pellitier L et al: Clinical assessment of the suicidal patient in the emergency department. JEN 10(1):40–43, 1984

Reubin R: Spotting and stopping the suicide patient. Nursing '79 9(4):82–85, 1979

Rigdon M: Death threat before and after attempted suicide: a clinical investigation. Death Educ 7(2–3):195–209, 1983

Rosenthal N: Death education and suicide potentiality. Death Educ 7(1):39–51, 1983

Seremet N: Needs of the attempted-suicide patient in the ICU. Crit Care Q 6(4):40–48, 1984

Talley J: Suicide prevention. On not being part of the problem. Consultant 23(6):33–37; 41, 1983

Valente S: Suicide in school aged children: theory and assessment. Pediatr Nurs 9(1):25–29, 1983

Zung W: Suicide prevention by suicide detection. Psychosomatics 20(3):149; 153–159, 1979

Suspiciousness

Articles

DiBella GAW: Educating staff to manage threatening paranoid patients. Am J Psychiatry 136(3):333–335, 1979

Tousley MM: The paranoid fortress of David J. J Psychosoc Nurs 22(2):8–16, 1984

Thought Processes, Alteration In

Articles

Knowles RD: Control your thoughts. Am J Nurs 81(2):353, 1981

Knowles RD: Disputing irrational thoughts. Am J Nurs 81(4):735, 1981

Schroder RJ: Nursing intervention with patient with thought disorders. Perspect Psychiatr Care 17(1):32–39, 1979

SELECTED NURSING INTERVENTIONS

Behavior Therapy

Books

Agras W (ed): Behavior Modification: Principles and Clinical Applications. Boston, Little, Brown, 1978

Banion D, Whaley D: Behavior Contracting: Arranging Contingencies of Reinforcement. New York, Springer-Verlag, 1981

Barker P: Behavior Therapy in Nursing. London, Croom Helm, 1982

Bellack A, Hersen M: Behavior Modification: An Introductory Textbook. Baltimore, Williams & Wilkins, 1977

Bellack A, Hersen M, Kazdin A (eds): International Handbook of Behavior Modification and Therapy. New York, Plenum Press, 1982

Berne E: Games People Play. The Psychology of Human Relationships. New York, Grove Press, 1966

Carr J, Yule W (eds): Behavior Modification for the Mentally Handicapped. Baltimore, University Park Press, 1980

Craig K, McMahon R (eds): Advances in Clinical Behavior Therapy. New York, Brunner/Mazel, 1983

Craighead W, Kazdin A, Mahoney M: Behavior Modification: Principles, Issues, and Applications. Boston, Houghton-Mifflin, 1981

Daitzman R (ed): Diagnosis and Intervention in Behavior Therapy and Behavioral Medicine. New York, Springer-Verlag, 1983

Fensterheim H, Glazer H: Behavioral Psychotherapy: Basic Principles and Case Studies in an Integrative Clinical Model. New York, Brunner/Mazel, 1983

Franks C (ed): New Developments in Behavior Therapy. New York, Haworth Press, 1984

Gelfand D, Hartmann D: Child Behavior Analysis and Therapy. New York, Pergamon Press, 1984

Goldstein A: Psychological Skill Training: The Structured Learning Technique. New York, Pergamon Press, 1981

Graziano A, Mooney K: Children and Behavior Therapy. New York, Aldine, 1984

Hall C: A Primer of Freudian Psychology. New York, New American Library, 1979

Hersen M (ed): Outpatient Behavior Therapy: A Clinical Guide. New York, Grune & Stratton, 1983

Hersen M, Bellack A (eds): Behavior Therapy in the Psychiatric Setting. Baltimore, Williams & Wilkins, 1978

Kazdin A: Behavior Modification in Applied Settings. Homewood, IL, Dorsey Press, 1975

Leitenberg H (ed): Handbook of Behavior Modification and Behavior Therapy. Englewood Cliffs, NJ, Prentice-Hall, 1976

Marks I: Care and Cure of Neuroses: Theory and Practice of Behavioral Psychotherapy. New York, John Wiley & Sons, 1981

Marmor J, Woods S (eds): The Interface Between the Psychodynamic and Behavioral Therapies. New York, Plenum Medical Book Co, 1980

Maultsky M: Rational Behavior Therapy. Englewood Cliffs, NJ, Prentice-Hall, 1984

May R: The Meaning of Anxiety. New York, W Norton, 1979

McMullin R, Giles T: Cognitive-Behavior Therapy: A Restructuring Approach. New York, Grune & Stratton, 1981

Quick E: Teaching Responsibility to Psychiatric Patients: A Behavioral-Humanistic Approach. Pittsburgh, Gateway Book Publishing Co, 1978

Rathus S, Nevid J: Behavior Therapy: Strategies for Solving Problems in Living. Garden City, Doubleday & Co, 1977

Reese E: The Analysis of Human Operant Behavior. Dubuque, Wm C. Brown, 1973

Reese E: Experiments in Operant Behavior. New York, Irvington, 1980

Rehm L: Behavior Therapy for Depression: Present Status and Future Directions. New York, Academic Press, 1980

Rosenbaum M, Franks C, Jaffe Y (eds): Perspectives on Behavior Therapy in the Eighties. New York, Springer-Verlag, 1983

Ross A: Child Behavior Therapy: Principles, Procedures, and Empirical Basis. New York, John Wiley & Sons, 1981

Spiegler M: Contemporary Behavioral Therapy. Palo Alto, Mayfield Publishing Co., 1983

Stolz S: Ethical Issues in Behavior Modification. San Francisco, Jossey-Bass, 1978

Whitman T, Scibak J, Reid D: Behavior Modification with the Severely and Profoundly Retarded. New York, Academic Press, 1983

Wilson G, Franks C (eds): Contemporary Behavior Therapy: Conceptual and Empirical Foundations. New York, Guilford Press, 1982

Wilson G, O'Leary K: Principles of Behavior Therapy. Englewood Cliffs, NJ, Prentice-Hall, 1980

Yates A: Biofeedback and the Modification of Behavior. New York, Plenum Press, 1980

Articles

Barker P: Behavior therapy in psychiatric and mental handicap nursing. J Adv Nurs 5(1):55–69, 1980

Butler R: The evolution of a token economy programme for female chronic schizophrenic patients. J Adv Nurs 4(3):307–318, 1979

Clark C: Combining therapeutic approaches. J Psychiatr Nurs 15(10):18–22, 1977

Hauser M: Nurses and behavior modification: resistance, ignorance or both. J Psychiatr Nurs 16(8):17–19, 1978

Mansdorf I, Bucich D, Judd L: Behavioral treatment strategies of institution ward staff. Ment Retard 15(5):22–24, 1977

Peterson K, Errickson E: Use of reinforcement principles to reinstate self-care activities in a deaf and blind psychiatric patient. J Psychiatr Nurs 15(6):15–18, 1977

Rumpler C, Seigerman C: A behavior modification approach to dealing with vio-

lent behavior in an intensive care unit. Perspect Psychiatr Care
16(5–6):206–211, 245, 1978

Schlemmer J, Barnett P: Management of manipulative behavior of anorexia ner-
vosa patients. J Psychiatr Nurs 15(11):35–41, 1977

Seidel H, Hodgkinson P: Behavior modification and long-term learning in Korsakoff's psychosis. Nurs Times 75(43):1855–1857, 1979

Weaver S, Armstrong N, Broome A et al: Behavioral principles applied in a security ward. Nurs Times 74(1):22–24, 1978

Group Therapy

Books

Aronson M, Wolberg L: Group and Family Therapy. New York, Brunner/Mazel,
1980

Benjamin A: Behavior in Small Groups. Boston, Houghton-Mifflin, 1978

Bion W: Experiences in Groups, and Other Papers. New York, Basic Books, 1961

Burnside I (ed): Working with the Elderly: Group Process and Techniques. Monterey, Wadsworth Health Sciences, 1984

Cartwright D, Zander A: Group Dynamics: Research and Theory. New York,
Harper & Row, 1968

Corey G, Corey M: Groups, Process and Practice. Monterey, Brooks/Cole Publishing Co, 1982

Dennis H: Remotivation therapy groups. In Burnside I (ed): Working with the
Elderly: Group Process and Techniques. North Scituate, Duxbury Press,
1978

Durkin J (ed): Living Groups: Group Psychotherapy and General System Theory.
New York, Brunner/Mazel, 1981

Ebersol P: Establishing reminiscing groups. In Burnside I (ed): Working with the
Elderly: Group Process and Techniques. North Scituate, Duxbury Press,
1978

Feder B, Ronall R (eds): Beyond the Hot Seat: Gestalt Approaches to Group. New
York, Brunner/Mazel, 1980

Gazda G (ed): Innovations to Group Psychotherapy. Springfield, IL, Charles C
Thomas, 1981

Gazda G (ed): Basic Approaches to Group Psychotherapy and Group Counseling.
Springfield, IL, Charles C Thomas, 1982

Grotjahn M, Kline F, Friedmann C: Handbook of Group Therapy. New York,
Van Nostrand Reinhold Co, 1983

Janosik E, Phipps L: Life Cycle Group Work in Nursing. Monterey, Wadsworth
Health Sciences Division, 1982

Kaplan H, Freedman A, Sadock B: Comprehensive Textbook of Psychiatry III.
Baltimore, Williams & Wilkins, 1980

Kaplan H, Sadock B (eds): Comprehensive Group Psychotherapy. Baltimore, Williams & Wilkins, 1983

Lennox D: Residential Group Therapy for Children. London, Tavistock, 1982

Lonergan E: Group Intervention, How to Begin and Maintain Groups in Medical
and Psychiatric Settings. New York, Aronson, 1982

Mullan H, Rosenbaum M: Group Psychotherapy: Theory and Practice. New
York, Free Press, 1978

Naar R: A Primer of Group Psychotherapy. New York, Human Sciences Press,
1982

Nickols M: Change in the Context of Group Therapy. New York, Brunner/Mazel,
1984

Oatley K: Selves in Relation: An Introduction to Psychotherapy and Groups. London, Methven, 1984

Paul G, Lentz R: Psychosocial Treatment of Chronic Mental Patients: Milieu Versus Social Learning Programs. Cambridge, Harvard University Press, 1979

Pines M, Rafaelsen L (eds): The Individual and the Group: Boundaries and Interrelations. New York, Plenum Press, 1982

Rose S: A Casebook in Group Therapy: A Behavioral Cognitive Approach. Englewood Cliffs, NJ, Prentice-Hall, 1980

Rosenbaum M (ed): Handbook of Short-Term Therapy Groups. New York, McGraw-Hill, 1983

Rosenfeld E: Group therapy. In Beck C, Rawlins R, Williams S (eds): Mental Health–Psychiatric Nursing. St Louis, CV Mosby, 1984

Rutan J, Stone W: Psychodynamic Group Psychotherapy. Lexington, MA, Collamore Press 1984

Sank L, Shaffer C: A Therapist's Manual for Cognitive Behavior Therapy in Groups. New York, Plenum Press, 1983

Schaefer C, Johnson L, Wherry J (eds): Group Therapies for Children and Youth. San Francisco, Jossey-Bass, 1982

Scheidlinger S: Focus on Group Psychotherapy: Clinical Essays. New York, International Universities Press, 1982

Schiffer M: Children's Group Therapy: Methods and Case Histories. New York, Free Press, 1984

Seligman M (ed): Group Psychotherapy and Counseling with Special Populations. Baltimore, University Park Press, 1982

Shapiro J: Methods of Group Psychotherapy and Encounter: A Tradition of Innovation. Itasca, FE Peacock Publishers, 1978

Slater P: Microcosm, Structural, Psychological, and Religious Evolution in Groups. New York, John Wiley & Sons, 1966

Starr A: Rehearsal for Living: Psychodrama. Chicago, Nelson Hall, 1977

Sullivan HS: The Interpersonal Theory of Psychiatry. New York, WW Norton, 1953

Taulbee L: Reality orientation: a therapeutic group activity for elderly persons. In Burnside I (ed): Working with the Elderly: Group Process and Techniques. North Scituate, Duxbury Press, 1978

Topalis M, Aguilera D: Psychiatric Nursing. St Louis, CV Mosby, 1978

Van Servellen G: Group and Family Therapy. St Louis, CV Mosby, 1984

Weiner M: Techniques of Group Psychotherapy. Washington DC, American Psychiatric Press, 1984

Wilson H, Kneisl C: Psychiatric Nursing. Menlo Park, CA, Addison-Wesley Publishing Co, 1983

Yablonsky L: Psychodrama. Resolving Emotional Problems Through Role-Playing. New York, Basic Books, 1976

Yalom I: Inpatient Group Psychotherapy. New York, Basic Books, 1983

Articles

Balgopal P, Vassil T: The group psychotherapist: a new breed. Perspect Psychiatr Care 17(3):132–135, 1979

Bennis W, Shepard H: A theory of group development. Hum Rel 9(4):415–437, 1956

Benton D: The significance of the absent member in milieu therapy. Perspect Psychiatr Care 18(1):21–25, 1980

Calicchia C, Governali J: Attitudes toward homosexuality: Does role-playing have an impact? Health Values 4(4):176–182, 1980

Cissna K: Phases in group development. Small Group Behavior 15(1):3–32, 1984

Frances A, Clarkin J, Marachi J: Selection criteria for outpatient group psychotherapy. Hosp Community Psychiatry 31(4):245–250, 1980

Hager R: Evaluation of group psychotherapy—a question of values. J Psychiatr Nurs 16(12):26, 31–33, 1978

Hankins-McNary L: The use of humor in group therapy. Perspect Psychiatr Care 17(5):228–231, 1979

Hardin S et al: The video connection: group dynamics on screen. J Psychosoc Nurs Ment Health Serv 21(11):12–17; 20–21, 1983

Hellwig K, Memmott R: Partners in therapy: using the co-therapists' relationship in a group. J Psychiatr Nurs 16(4):42–44, 1978

Horowitz J: Sexual difficulties as indicators of broader personal and interpersonal problems. Perspect Psychiatr Care 16(2):66–69, 1978

Janosik E: Reachable and teachable: report on a prison alcoholism group. J Psychiatr Nurs 15(4):24–28, 1977

Jordan T: Group process in action—a detoxification unit for alcoholics. Free Assoc 10(3):7–8; 10, 1983

Kiernat J: The use of life review activity with confused nursing home residents. Am J Occup Ther 33(5):306–310, 1979

Lyon G: Stimulation through remotivation. Am J Nurs 71(5):982–985, 1971

Matteson M et al: Group reminiscing therapy with elderly clients. Issues Ment Health Nurs 4(3):177–189, 1982

McIvor D, Rosario A: Group therapy for women going through divorce. Can J Psychiatr Nurs 20(3):11–13, 1979

McMordie W, Blom S: Life review therapy: psychotherapy for the elderly. Perspect Psychiatr Care 17(4):162–166, 1979

Neizo B et al: Medication groups on an acute psychiatric unit. Perspect Psychiatr Care 21(2):70–73, 1983

Pullinger W: Remotivation. Am J Nurs 60(5):682–685, 1960

Rioch M: The work of Wilfred Bion on groups. Psychiatry 33(1):56–66, 1970

Sanderson M, Blackley J: Problems displayed "in vivo"—a particular advantage of group therapy. Perspect Psychiatr Care 17(4):176–186, 1979

Slimmer L: Use of the nursing process to facilitate group therapy. J Psychiatr Nurs 16(2):42–44, 1978

Smith L: Finding your leadership style in groups. Am J Nurs 80(7):1301–1303, 1980

Stryker R: How to develop a therapeutic community. J Nurs Adm 10(4):14–17, 1980

Tappen R et al: Group leader—Are you a controller? J Gerontol Nurs 9(1):34–38; 44; 59, 1983

Wise P: Methods of teaching—revisited character play and role play. J Cont Ed Nurs 11(1):37–38, 1980

Wynne A: Movable group therapy for institutionalized patients. Hosp Community Psychiatry 29(8):516–519, 1978

Administration of Drug Therapy

Books

Albanese JA: Nurses' Drug Reference, 2nd ed. New York, McGraw-Hill, 1982

Bernstein JG: Handbook of Drug Therapy in Psychiatry. Boston, John Wright, 1983

Czáky TZ, Barnes BA: Cutting's Handbook of Pharmacology, 7th ed. Norwalk, CT, Appleton-Century-Crofts, 1984

Gilman AG, Goodman LS, Gilman A (eds): Goodman and Gilman's the Pharmacological Basis of Therapeutics, 6th ed. New York, Macmillan, 1980

Govoni LE, Hayes JE: Drugs and Nursing Implications, 4th ed. Norwalk, CT, Appleton-Century-Crofts, 1982

Jeste DV, Wyatt RJ: Understanding and Treating Tardive Dyskinesia. New York, Guilford Press, 1982

Klein DF, Gittelman R, Quitkin F, Rifkin A: Diagnosis and Drug Treatment of Psychiatric Disorders: Adults and Children, 2nd ed. Baltimore, Williams & Wilkins, 1980

Loebl S, Spratto G, Heckheimer E: The Nurse's Drug Handbook, 3rd ed. New York, John Wiley & Sons, 1983

Physicians' Desk Reference, 37th edition. New Jersey, Medical Economics, 1983

Schon M: Lithium Treatment of Manic-Depressive Illness. A Practical Guide. Basel, S Karger International, 1980

Sheridan E, Patterson HR, Gustafson EA: Falcomer's the Drug, the Nurse, the Patient, 7th ed. Philadelphia, WB Saunders, 1982

Spencer RT et al: Clinical Pharmacology and Nursing Management. Philadelphia JB Lippincott, 1983

United States Pharmacopeial Convention, Inc. About Your Medicines. Kingsport, TN, Kingsport Press, 1982

Van Praag HM (ed): Handbook of Biological Psychiatry. Part V. Drugs in Psychiatry-Psychotropic Drugs. New York, Marcel Dekker, 1981

Wilson HS, Kneisl CR: Psychiatric Nursing, 2nd ed. Menlo Park, CA, Addison-Wesley Publishing, Co, 1983

Articles

Blackwell B: Antidepressant drugs: Side effects and compliance. J Clin Psychiatry 43(11):14–18, 1982

Boettcher EG, Alderson SF: Psychotropic medications and the nursing process. J Psychosocial Nurs Ment Health Serv 20(11):12–16, 1982

Cohen M, Amdur MA: Medication group for psychiatric patients. Am J Nurs 81(2):343–345, 1981

Cohen M, Gordon R, Marlowe H et al: A single-bedtime-dose self-medication system. Hosp Community Psychiatry 30(1):30–33, 1979

DeGennaro MD, Hymen R, Crannell AM, Mansky PA: Antidepressant drug therapy. Am J Nurs 81(7):1304–1310, 1981

Ereshefsky L et al: Future of depot neuroleptic therapy: pharmacokinetic and pharmacodynamic approaches. J Clin Psychiatry 45(5):50–59, 1984

Feldman J, Wilner S, Winickoff R: A study of lithium carbonate use in a health maintenance organization. QRB 8(9):8–14, 1982

Gever LN: Anticholinergics. Nursing '84 14(9):64: 1984

Ghadirian AM, Lehnann HE: Neurological side effects of lithium: organic brain syndrome, seizures; extrapyramidal side effects, and EEG changes. Compr Psychiatry 21(5):327–334, 1980

Harris E: Antipsychotic medications. Am J Nurs 81(7):1316–1323, 1981

Harris E: Extrapyramidal side effects of antipsychotic medications. Am J Nurs 81(7):1324–1328, 1981

Harris E: Lithium. Am J Nurs 81(7):1310–1315, 1981

Harris E: Sedative-hypnotic drugs. Am J Nurs 81(7):1329–1334, 1981

Jamison KR, Akiskal HS: Medication compliance in patients with bipolar disorder. Psychiatr Clin North Am 6(1):175–192, 1983

Jefferson JW et al: Effect of strenuous exercise on serum lithium level in man. Am J Psychiatry 139(12):1593–1595, 1982

Kessler KA, Waletzky JP: Clinical use of the antipsychotics. Am J Psychiatry 139(2):202–209, 1981

Larkin AL: What's a medication group? J Psychosocial Nurs Ment Health Serv 20(2):35–37, 1982

Manoquerra AS: Tricyclic antidepressants. Crit Care Q 4(4):43–54, 1982

Mann SC, Boger WP: Psychotropic drugs, summer heat and humidity, and hyperpyrexia: a danger restated. Am J Psychiatry 135(9):1097–1100, 1978

Mason AS, Granacher RP: Basic principles of rapid neuroleptization. Dis Nerv Syst 37(10):547–551, 1976

Neizo B, Murphy MK: Medication groups on an acute psychiatric unit. Perspect Psychiatr Care 21(2):70–73, 1983

Rosal-Greif VLF: Drug-induced dyskinesias. Am J Nurs 82(1):66–69, 1982

Schou M, Vestergaard P: Lithium and the kidney scare (editorial). Psychosomatics 22(2):92; 94, 1981

Settle EC, Ayd FJ: Haloperidol: a quarter century of experience. J Clin Psychiatry 44(12):440–448, 1983

Smith JE: Improving drug knowledge in psychiatric patients. J Psychosocial Nurs Ment Health Serv 19(4):16–18, 1981

Task force on late neurological effects of antipsychotic drugs. Am J Psychiatry 137(10):1163–1172, 1980

Van Putten T, May PRA, Marder SR: Response to antipsychotic medication: the doctor's and the consumer's view. Am J Psychiatry 141(1):16–19, 1984

Vestergaard P: Clinically important side effects of long-term lithium treatment: a review. Acta Psychiatr Scand (Suppl) 305:1–36, 1983

Whall AL et al: Development of a screening program for tardive dyskinesia: Feasibility issues. Nurs Res 32(3):151–156, 1983

Whiteside SE: Patient education: effectiveness of medication programs for psychiatric patients. J Psychosocial Nurs Ment Health Serv 21(10):16–21, 1983

Zubenko G, Pope HG: Management of a case of neuroleptic malignant syndrome with bromocriptine. Am J Psychiatry 140(12):1619–1620, 1983

Pamphlet

National Institute of Mental Health and the Office of Medical Applications of Research: Mood Disorders: Pharmacologic prevention of recurrences. Consensus Development Conference, April 24–26, 1984

Protective Interventions

Books

Albert HD: Specific technics with dangerous or armed patients. In Stone MH et al (eds): Treating Schizophrenic Patients, a Clinico-Analytical Approach. New York, McGraw-Hill, 1983

Blake K, Taylor EC: The Prevention and Management of Aggressive Behavior. Columbia, SC, Department of Mental Health, 1977

Murray RB, Huelskoetter MM: Psychiatric/Mental Health Nursing, Giving Emotional Care. Englewood Cliffs, NJ, Prentice-Hall, 1983

Articles

Bell CC, Palmer JM: Security procedures in a psychiatric emergency service. J Natl Med Assoc 73(9):835–842, 1981

Binder RL, McCoy SM: A study of patients' attitudes toward placement in seclusion. Hosp Community Psychiatry 34(11):1052–1054, 1983

Blythe MM, Pearlmutter DR: The suicide watch: a re-examination of maximum observation. Perspect Psychiatr Care 21(3):90–93, 1983

Busteed EL, Johnstone C: The development of suicide precautions for an inpatient psychiatric unit. J Psychosocial Nurs Ment Health Serv 21(5):15–19, 1983

Capodanno AE, Targum SD: Assessment of suicide risk: some limitations in the infrequent events. J Psychosocial Nurs Ment Health Serv 21(5):11–14, 1983

DiBella GA: Educating staff to manage threatening paranoid patients. Am J Psychiatry 136(3):333–335, 1979

Gerlock A, Solomons HC: Factors associated with the seclusion of psychiatric patients. Perspect Psychiatr Care 21(2):46–53, 1983

Gertz B: Training for prevention of assaultive behavior in a psychiatric setting. Hosp Community Psychiatry 31(9):628–630, 1980

Gutheil TG, Daly M: Clinical considerations in seclusion room design. Hosp Community Psychiatry 31(4):268–270, 1980

Hoff LA, Resing M: Was this suicide preventable? Am J Nurs 82(7):1106–1111, 1982

Jacobs D: Evaluation and management of the violent patient in emergency settings. Psychiatr Clin North Am 6(2):259–269, 1983

Maagdenberg AM: The violent patient. Am J Nurs 83(3):402–403, 1983

McCoy SM, Garritson S: Seclusion: the process of intervening. J Psychosocial Nurs Ment Health Serv 21(8):9–15, 1983

Oldham JM, Russakoff LM, Prusnofsky L: Seclusion: patterns and milieu. J Nerv Ment Dis 171(11):645–650, 1983

Phillips MA, Nasr SJ: Seclusion and restraint and prediction of violence. Am J Psychiatry 140(2):229–232, 1983

Redmond FC: Study on the use of the seclusion room. QRB 6(8):20–32, 1980

Rosen H, Dibiacomo J: The role of physical restraint in the treatment of psychiatric illness. J Clin Psychiatry 39(3):228–232, 1978

Soloff PH, Turner SM: Patterns of seclusion, a prospective study. J Nerv Ment Dis 169(1):37–44, 1981

MAJOR PSYCHIATRIC DISORDERS

Books

Aguilera AC, Mesnick JM: Crisis Intervention Theory and Methodology, 4th ed. St Louis, CV Mosby, 1982

American Psychiatric Association: Electroconvulsive Therapy. Task Force Report No. 14. Washington DC, American Psychiatric Association, 1978

American Psychiatric Association: Diagnostic and Statistical Manual of Mental Disorders, 3rd ed. Washington DC, American Psychiatric Association, 1980

Arieti S: The Intrapsychic Self. New York, Basic Books, 1967

Arieti S, Bemporad J: Severe and Mild Depression. New York, Basic Books, 1978

Barofsky I, Budson RD: The Chronic Psychiatric Patient in the Community: Principles of Treatment. New York, Spectrum Publishing, 1983

Basmajian JV (ed): Biofeedback, Principles and Practice for Clinicians, 2nd ed. Baltimore, Williams & Wilkins, 1983

Beck AT: Cognitive Therapy and Emotional Disorders. New York, International Universities Press, 1976

Blatner HA: Acting-In. Practical Applications of Psychodramatic Methods. New York, Springer-Verlag, 1973

Bootzin RR, Acocella JR: Abnormal Psychology: Current Perspective. New York, Random House, 1984

Bowen M: Family Therapy and Clinical Practice. New York, Jason-Aroson, 1978

Burns DD: Feeling Good, The New Mood Therapy. New York, William Morrow, 1980

Chambers DG, Goldstein AJ (eds): Agoraphobia, Multiple Perspectives on Therapy and Treatment. New York, John Wiley & Sons, 1982

Cole JO, Schatzberg AF, Frazier SH (eds): Depression: Biology, Psychodynamics, and Treatment. New York, Plenum Press, 1978

Davis M et al: The Relaxation and Stress Reduction Workbook, 2nd ed. Richmond, CA, New Harbinger, 1982

Ellis A, Harper RA: A New Guide to Rational Living. Englewood Cliffs, NJ, Prentice-Hall, 1975

Emmelkamp PMG: Phobic and Obsessive-Compulsive Disorders, Theory, Research and Practice. New York, Plenum Press, 1982

Folsom JC: Reality orientation. In Resiberg B (ed): Alzheimer's Disease. New York, Free Press, 1983

Ford DH, Urban HB: Systems of Psychotherapy. New York, John Wiley & Sons, 1963

Gaines J: Fritz Perls, Here and Now. Milbrae, CA, Celestial Arts, 1979

Gelder M, Gath D, Mayou R: Oxford Textbook of Psychiatry. Oxford, Oxford University Press, 1983

Glaser W: Mental Health or Mental Illness: Psychiatry for Practical Action. New York, Harper & Row, 1983

Glaser W: Take Effective Control of Your Life. New York, Harper & Row, 1984

Greenberg IA (ed): Psychodrama, Theory and Therapy. New York, Behavior Publications, 1974

Guerin PJ (ed): Family Therapy, Theory and Practice. New York, Gardner Press, 1976

Hatcher C, Milstein P (eds): The Handbook of Gestalt Therapy. New York, Aronson, 1976

Heston LL, White JA: Dementia: A Practical Guide to Alzheimer's Disease and Related Illnesses. New York, WH Freeman & Co, 1983

Hopkins HL, Smith HD (eds): Willard and Spackman's Occupational Therapy, 6th ed. Philadelphia, JB Lippincott, 1983

Hyde AP: Living with Schizophrenia. Chicago, Contemporary Books, 1980

Jellinek EM: Phases in the Drinking History of Alcoholics. New Haven, CT, Hillhouse Press, 1946

Kaplan HI, Freedman AM, Sadock BJ (eds): Comprehensive Textbook of Psychiatry, Vol II, 3rd ed. Baltimore, Williams & Wilkins, 1980

Kimble GA, Garmezy N, Zigler E: Principles of Psychology, 6th ed. New York, John Wiley & Sons, 1984

Klein M: Lives People Live: A Textbook of Transactional Analysis. New York, John Wiley & Sons, 1980

Klerman G, Weissman M: Interpersonal Psychotherapy of Depression. New York, Basic Books, 1984

Kolb LC, Brodie HK: Modern Clinical Psychiatry, 10th ed. Philadelphia, WB Saunders, 1982

Lewinsohn P, Teri L (eds): Coping and Adaptation in the Elderly. New York, Pergamon Press, 1983

Lishman W: Organic Psychiatry. London, Blackwell Scientific Publications, 1978

Meissner WW: The Borderline Spectrum: Differential Diagnosis and Developmental Issues. New York, Jason Aronson, 1984

Miller JD, Cisin IH: Highlights From the National Survey on Drug Abuse, 1982. DHHS Pub. No. (ADM)83-1277. Rockville, MD, National Institute on Drug Abuse, 1983

Miller W (ed): The Addictive Behaviors: Treatment of Alcoholism, Drug Abuse, Smoking and Obesity. New York, Pergamon Press, 1980

Minuchin S: Families and Family Therapy. Cambridge, MA, Harvard University Press, 1974

Moreno JL: Psychodrama. New York, Beacon House, 1945

Morgan WP: Physical activity and mental health. In Eckert HM, Montoye HJ (eds). Exercise and Health. Champaign, IL, Human Kinetics, 1984

Nadelson CC, Marcotte DB: Treatment Interventions in Human Sexuality. In Nadelson CC, Marcotte DB (eds). Critical Issues in Psychiatry. New York, Plenum Press, 1983

Pardeck JA, Pardeck JT: Young People with Problems: A Guide to Bibliotherapy. Westport, CT, Greenwood Press, 1984

Peterfreund E: The Process of Psychoanalytic Therapy, Models & Strategies. Hillsdale, NJ, The Analytic Press, 1983

Reed KL: Models of Practice in Occupational Therapy. Baltimore, Williams & Wilkins, 1984

Reisberg B (ed): Alzheimer's Disease. New York, Free Press, 1983

Rogers C: Freedom to Learn. Vermont, Merrill, 1982

Shapiro SA: Contemporary Theories of Schizophrenia: Review and Synthesis. New York, McGraw-Hill, 1981

Siesel EV: The Mirror of Ourselves: A Psychoanalytic Approach. New York, Human Sciences Press, 1984

Statistical Compendium in Alcohol and Health: DHHS Pub. No. (ADM)81-1115. Rockville, MD, National Institute on Alcohol Abuse and Alcoholism, 1981

Stone MH et al: Treating Schizophrenic Patients, A Clinico-analytical Approach. New York, McGraw-Hill, 1983

Sullivan HS: Interpersonal Theory of Psychiatry. New York, WW Norton, 1953

Tabakoff B, Stuker PB, Randall CL (eds): Medical and Social Aspects of Alcohol Abuse. New York, Plenum Press, 1983

Thorpe GL, Burns LE: The Agoraphobic Syndrome, Behavorial Approaches to Evaluation and Treatment. New York, John Wiley & Sons, 1983

Turner F (ed): Adult Psychopathology: A Social Work Perspective. New York, Free Press, 1984

Williams JMG: The Psychological Treatment of Depression: A Guide to the Theory and Practice of Cognitive-Behavior Therapy. London, Croom Helm, 1984

Yalom ID: The Theory and Practice of Group Psychotherapy, 2nd ed. New York, Basic Books, 1975

Articles

Ahern L: Electroconvulsive therapy: an effective treatment. ADRNJ 34(3):463-470, 1981

Beam IM: Helping families survive. Am J Nurs 84(2):229-232, 1984

Beels CC, McFarlane WR: Family treatments of schizophrenia: background and state of the art. Hosp Community Psychiatry 33(7):541-550, 1982

Berkowitz R, Heinl P: The management of schizophrenic patients: the nurses' view. J Adv Nurs 9(1):23-34, 1984

Berner J, Earnest MP: Alcohol withdrawal syndromes. Top Emerg Med
6(2):39–47, 1984

Betemps E: Management of the withdrawal syndrome of barbiturates and other
central nervous system depressants. J Psychosoc Nurs Ment Health Serv
19(9):31–34, 1981

Bowman C, Spadoni AJ: Assertion therapy: the nurse and the psychiatric patient
in an acute, short-term hospital setting. J Psychosoc Nurs Ment Health Serv
19(6):1–21, 1981

Boyd JH, Weissman MM: Epidemiology of affective disorders. Arch Gen Psychiatry 38(9):1039–1046, 1981

Brady JP: Social skills training for psychiatric patients, I: Concepts, methods, and
clinical results. Am J Psychiatry 141(3):333–340, 1984

Brady JP: Social skills training for psychiatric patients, II: Clinical outcome studies. Am J Psychiatry 141(4):491–498, 1984

Breier A, Charney DS, Heninger GR: Major depression in patients with agoraphobia and panic disorder. Arch Gen Psychiatry 41(12):1129–1135, 1984

Brier A, Strauss JS: The role of social relationships in the recovery from psychotic
disorders. Am J Psychiatry 141(8):949–955, 1984

Brodsley L: Avoiding a crisis: the assessment. Am J Nurs 82(12):1865–1871,
1982

Chaisson M et al: Treating the depressed elderly. J Psychosocial Nurs Ment
Health Serv 22(5):25–30, 1984

Cochran C: A change of mind. Am J Nurs 84(8):1004–1005, 1984

Cohn L: The hidden diagnosis. Am J Nurs 82(12):1862–1864, 1982

Coyne JC, Gotlib IH: The role of cognition in depression: a critical appraisal. Psychol Bull 94(3):472–505, 1983

Crowe RR: Electroconvulsive therapy: a current perspective. N Engl J Med
311(3):163–167, 1984

Danziger S: Major treatment issues and techniques in family therapy with the
borderline adolescent. J Psychosoc Ment Health Nurs 20(1):27–34, 1982

Dimotto JW: Relaxation. Am J Nurs 84(6):754–758, 1984

Dixson DL: Manic depression: an overview. J Psychosoc Nurs Ment Health Serv
19(6):28–31, 1981

Docherry JP et al: Stages of onset of schizophrenic psychosis. Am J Psychiatry
135(4):420–426, 1978

Efinger JM: Women and alcoholism. Top Clin Nurs 4(4):10–19, 1983

Falloon RH et al: Family management in the prevention of exacerbations of
schizophrenia, a controlled study. N Engl J Med 306(24):1438–1440,
1982

Fishel AH, Jefferson CB: Assertiveness training for hospitalized, emotionally disturbed women. Psychosoc Nurs Ment Health Serv 21(11):22–27, 1983

Gordon G, Beresin E: Conflicting models for inpatient management of borderline
patients. Am J Psychiatry 140(8):979–983, 1983

Groves JE: Current concepts in psychiatry: borderline personality disorder. N Engl
Med J 305(5):259–262, 1981

Herz MI: Recognizing and preventing relapse in patients with schizophrenia.
Hosp Community Psychiatry 35(4):344–349, 1984

Hollace S, Mittleman RE, Mittleman BE: Cocaine. Am J Nurs 84(9):1092–1095,
1984

Kahn EM: Psychotherapy with chronic schizophrenics: alliance, transference,
and countertransference. J Psychosoc Nurs Ment Health Serv 22(7):20–25,
1984

Keisling R: Underdiagnosis of manic-depressive illness in a hospital unit. Am J Psychiatry 138(5):672–673, 1981

Krenzelok EP: Phencyclidine—a contemporary drug of abuse. Crit Care Q 4(4):55–63, 1982

Kurose K et al: A standard care plan for alcoholism. Am J Nur 81(5):1001–1006, 1981

Leporati NC, Chychula LH: How you can really help the drug-abusing patient. Nursing 12(6):46–49, 1982

Lloyd C: Life events and depressive disorder reviewed: 1. Events as predisposing factors. Arch Gen Psychiatry 37(5):529–535, 1980

Marx JA, Bar-Or D: Wernike-Korsakoff syndrome. Top Emerg Med 6(2):83–87, 1984

Mattes JA: The optimal length of hospitalization for psychiatric patients: a review of the literature. Hosp Community Psychiatry 33(10):824–828, 1982

McCoy S, Rice MJ, McFadden K: PCP intoxication: psychiatric issues of nursing care. J Psychosoc Nurs Ment Health Serv 19(7):17–23, 1981

Morell MA, Levine M, Perkins DV: Study of behavioral factors associated with psychiatric rehospitalization. Community Ment Health J 18(3):190–199, 1982

Nadi S, Nurnberger JI, Gershon ES: Muscarinic cholinergic receptors in skin fibroblasts in familial affective disorder. N Engl J Med 311(4):225–230, 1984

Newton G: Self-help groups: Can they help? J Psychosoc Nurs Ment Health Serv 22(7):27–31, 1984

Pajk M: Inpatient care. Am J Nurs 84(2):215–222, 1984

Pallikkathayil L, Tweed S: Substance abuse: alcohol and drugs during adolescence. Nurs Clin North Am 18(2):313–321, 1983

Platt-Kock LM: Borderline personality disorder: a therapeutic approach. Am J Nurs 83(12):1666–1671, 1983

Pyke J, Page J: Schizophrenia. Can Nurs 77(5):39–43, 1981

Pyke J, Page J: Long-term care for the chronic schizophrenic patient. Can Nurs 78(1):37–44, 1982

Reisberg B: Stages of cognitive decline. Am J Nurs 84(2):225–228, 1984

Reisberg B, Ferris SH: Diagnosis and assessment of the older patient. Hosp Community Psychiatry 33(2):104–110, 1982

Richardson K: Hope and flexibility: your keys to helping OBS patients. Nursing 12(6):65–69, 1982

Roberts CM: RET: Rational/emotional therapy—a cognitive-behavior treatment system. Perspect Psychiatr Care 20(3):134–138, 1982

Scherwerts P: An alcoholic treatment team. Am J Nurs 82(12):1878–1879, 1982

Schloemer NF, Skidmore JW: Opiate withdrawal and clonidine. J Psychosocial Nurs Ment Health Serv 21(10):8–14, 1983

Siegel J, Scipio-Skinner KV: Psychodrama: an experiential model for nursing students. J Group Psychother Psychodrama Sociometry 36(3):97–101, 1983

Slavinsky AT, Krauss JB: Two approaches to the management of long-term psychiatric outpatients in the community. Nurs Res 31(5):284–289, 1982

Teusink JP, Mahler S: Helping families cope with Alzheimer's disease. Hosp Community Psychiatry 35(2):152–156, 1984

Theories and therapies. Am J Nurs 84(2):223–224, 1984

Weiner RD: The psychiatric use of electrically induced seizures. Am J Psychiatry 136(12):1507–1517, 1979

Weist JK, Lindeman MG, Newton M: Hospital dialogues. Am J Nurs 82(12):1874–1877, 1982

Wells CE: Chronic brain disease: an overview. Am J Psychiatry 135(1):1–10, 1978

Zyl SV: Psychotherapy with the elderly. J Psychosoc Nurs Ment Health Serv 21(10):25–29, 1983

Pamphlet

Goodwin FK: Depression and Manic Depressive Illness. NIH Pub. No. 82-1940. Bethesda, MD, National Institutes of Health, February, 1982

Index

Numbers followed by an *f* indicate a figure; *n* following a page number indicates footnoted material; *t* following a page number indicates tabular material.

abstract thinking, assessment of, 36
abuse, defined, 177. *See also* alcohol
    abuse; drug abuse
acceptance
    in grieving, 78, 80
    in therapeutic relationship, 25–26
acetophenazine (Tindal), 150t
acetylcholine, 3, 4
action
    in adaptive strategy, 27
    assessment of, 32–33
active listening, 21
activity reinforcers, 141
activity therapy, 201
adaptation
    in conceptual framework for psychi-
        atric nursing practice, 27
    to stress, 5–6
addiction, to drugs, 122. *See also* drug
    abuse
adjunctive groups, 142
affective disorders
    clinical manifestations of, 191–192
    defined, 190
    etiology of, 191
    health education for, 192
    incidence of, 190–191
    nursing diagnoses with, 192–193
    treatment of, 192
affective state
    assessment of, 36–37
    in delirium, 173
affective syndrome, organic, 174
affective words, patient's use of, 18

aggression, inappropriate
    defined, 44
    defining characteristics of, 45–46
    etiology of, 44–45
    evaluation/outcome criteria for, 50
    general principles for, 44
    goals and nursing interventions for,
        47–50
    health education and prevention
        for, 50
    model of, 45t
    nursing assessment of, 46–47
aggressive drive, 6
agranulocytosis, 154
akathesia, 153
akinesia, 153
Akineton (biperiden), 164t
alcohol abuse
    clinical manifestations of, 180–181
    defined, 116
    defining characteristics of, 117–118
    etiology of, 116–117, 178
    evaluation/outcome criteria for, 121
    general principles for, 116
    goals and nursing interventions for,
        118–120
    health education and prevention
        for, 120–121, 184
    incidence of, 177–178
    nursing assessment of, 118
    nursing diagnoses associated with,
        184–185
    treatment of, 182–184
Alcoholics Anonymous, 183